^{THE} Act_{*of*}
LIVING

WALTER CARRINGTON

THE
Act *of*
TALKS ON THE ALEXANDER TECHNIQUE
LIVING

EDITED BY JERRY SONTAG

MORNUM TIME PRESS

© 1999 Walter Carrington

Second Printing, 2004
Third Printing, 2008.

Printed, bound and published in the United States of America by
Mornum Time Press

To order additional copies, send $32.50 (postpaid) to Mornum Time
Press, 682 Santa Barbara Road, Berkeley, California 94707.

Text and cover design by Marianne Ackerman, 12 Haumia Street,
Paekakariki, New Zealand.

Library of Congress Catalog Card Number: 99-70477

ISBN 0-9644352-3-3

Contents

Foreword IX

Author's preface XXI

Editor's note XXIII

Introduction XXVII

Thinking to do 1

General functioning 7

Habits of thought and action 11

Sciatica 15

What you don't want 19

Taking the pressure off 23

The feet 29

The balance of the head 33

The length and the width 39

Coordinated use 43

The mechanics of the situation 47

Apart from all knowledge   55

A visual impression   61

Theory and practice   67

Spinal curvature   71

The primary wish   77

Forward and up   81

Knees forward and away   89

Walking   97

Everything flows   101

Working the wheel   107

Yin and yang   113

Establishing a total pattern   119

Responsibility   125

Gravitation   129

Saying and meaning no   135

A sense of insecurity   141

Change without changing   145

The act of living   149

Biographies

Foreword

IT IS NOW OVER FORTY YEARS since my
first contact with the Alexander Technique. A friend of
mine who is a professional musician had taken lessons
from Charles Neil at Lansdowne Road, then called the
"Isobel Cripps Centre." I visited the Centre and had a
long and friendly talk with Charles. I formed the opinion
that there was nothing in the Technique that was out of
line with orthodox neurophysiology, though the language was very different. The differences appeared more
marked when I came to read Alexander's writings. In
particular, I felt that the word "inhibition" was being
used incorrectly. Etymologically, the word suggests
restraint, that is to say, interference with what would otherwise happen. Thus the sense used by chemists and
physiologists may be stated in the following fashion: "If a
situation A is commonly followed by B, so long as C is
not present, then we say that C inhibits the response B to
A." The absence of B when A is not present does not, of
itself, imply the action of any inhibitory process. I felt
that, in the Alexander context, the expression "refraining
from action" might be more appropriate.

It was only some years later, when I met Walter Carrington, and he had given me a demonstration, that I started to wonder just what it is that the teacher is doing to his client. In this book, Walter doesn't use any of the jargon of science, preferring the locutions of common speech, so that his discourse is accessible to anyone, whatever their background. He does, however, use a few expressions which are familiar only to those already exposed to Alexander's writings. This is appropriate since the text consists of transcripts of tapes of talks to aspiring teachers of the Technique. The occasional use of such expressions should not, however, seriously interfere with understanding for the ordinary reader.

The general problem with jargon is that, when the initiated look for a short-hand expression to refer to a familiar but complex situation, there is a great temptation to use ordinary words as labels rather than in their generally accepted meaning. As an example, we may take the jargon use of expressions such as "going up" or "pulling down." In the Alexander context, "going up" does not necessarily imply movement, and "pulling down" needs to be interpreted carefully in relation to the mechanics of muscular action, as I shall explain later.

The up/down direction is usually taken as determined by the gravitational vertical but, as I explain in some detail in my book *Understanding Balance*, the situation is by no means so simple as at first appears. The "behavioural vertical," which is the direction that is used by the body in practice when organising the musculature for the purpose of maintaining balance, depends on a complex process of judgment that takes account of a great many factors, such as whether one is supported on a stationary base, such as the ground, or is in a moving vehicle, especially one which is accelerating, and whether one wishes to stay in the same place or to move around. The "gravitational vertical," i.e the direction of the gravitational field, is seldom relevant.

The core of the difficulty lies in Newton's use of the word *gravitas*. He was writing in Latin, which was the language of science in his day. The Latin language has a much more restricted vocabulary, in comparison with the very much richer vocabulary we are accustomed to in English. In Latin, nuances of meaning are indicated by context and word order, whereas, in English we often use separate words to convey subtle distinctions of meaning. Before Newton's time, the word *gravitas* indicated the property of being heavy, of requiring effort to lift the object. Another property is that, in the ordinary terrestrial environment, objects fall if they are not supported, and ingenious experiments are required to measure the speed of falling.

Newton continued Gallileo's experiments with the trajectories of spheres rolling across inclined planes and confirmed that the downward acceleration was independent of the size or weight of the spheres. He had already formulated his first two Laws of Motion, setting out what is to be understood by the word "force," and how it was to be measured, as the "rate of change of momentum." This led him to conclude that falling objects are subjected to a force. He was most unhappy with this conclusion since such a force was clearly able to exert its influence without contact, in contrast to all the other instances then known of the action of forces, which depended on contact between objects. He delayed publication of his conclusion for about twenty years, but continued to use the word *gravitas* both for heaviness and for the force accelerating unsupported objects. Meanwhile he extended the application of this new idea until he had established that it provided an extraordinarily precise way of describing the motions of the heavenly bodies.

We are nowadays much more familiar with the notion of field effects, from the development of the physics of molecular, atomic and nuclear structures. The forces of common experience, of pushing and pulling, adhesion and elasticity, all turn out to be manifestations, on a domestic scale, of the complex web of interacting field forces in and between molecules. Physicists tend, now, to pay more attention to field forces and leave effects on the domestic scale, such as stress and strain, to the engineers. We now use "gravity" mostly in the sense of Newton's force acting at a distance, but the older sense of *gravitas* is still preserved in terms such as "centre of gravity" and "specific gravity," which are to do with heaviness rather than with Newtonian gravity.

This leads to confusion when dealing with concepts such as "weight," which is related to "heaviness" in rather a subtle fashion. Heaviness is to do with stress, which involves deformation of molecular architecture, manifested as "strain." When we wish to assess the "weight" of an object we may use either a beam balance or a spring balance. A beam balance provides a comparison between objects placed in the two pans, since the two pans tend to tilt the beam in opposite directions, while a spring balance depends on measuring the strain in a deformable spring used to support the object to be weighed, with calibration depending again on a comparison between the deflections associated with different objects. Both measuring devices need to be "at rest" when the measurements are taken, and both are equally dependent on the stress forces needed to support objects in a scale pan. When we assess the weight of something held in the hand, it is the detection of strain in parts of the body that is used to develop our assessment.

Stress can be detected by measuring the accompanying strain, or deformation, because the association of stress with strain is a fundamental property of the interaction between molecules by short-range forces. Gravity, in the Newtonian sense, cannot be detected directly. It is only inferred from its effects, i.e. by the associated acceleration. For objects that are stationary with respect to the earth's surface we suppose that the action of Newtonian gravity is unaffected by the fact that the objects are sup-

ported, and that the supporting forces combine to produce an upward acceleration equal and opposite to that
attributable to Newtonian gravity. We measure the strain
associated with the supporting forces and this gives us an
indirect measure of the force of gravity in those conditions. It must be remembered that this argument is valid
only for objects that are at rest on the surface of the earth
or are supported by other structures that are also at rest
on the earth's surface. Gravity and stress do not oppose
one another, as is often supposed, but act simultaneously,
each producing its own acceleration. That these accelera-
tions are not necessarily equal is seen clearly during running and jumping, especially in jumping from a
trampoline, since there is no supporting force during the
flight phase, while gravity continues unabated and is
responsible for the downward return towards the earth.
The conditions in an orbiting spacecraft, after the rocket
propulsion has been switched off, are precisely the same
as those during the flight phase of a jump. The notion
that gravity ceases to act during the free fall phase, to
produce a state of so-called "zero gravity," is clearly
incorrect if "gravity" is taken in the Newtonian sense.
What is missing is the "heaviness," since there is no need
for stress forces to keep objects in place within the cap-
sule, because this is, itself, also in free fall and accelerating
towards the earth under the action of gravity.

Another consideration to keep in mind in relation to
stress forces is that they always act in two directions: the

forces supporting an object push upwards against the object and, at the same time, push downward against the supports. This essential property of stress forces is expressed in Newton's Third Law: "To every force there is an equal and opposite reaction force." Newton assumed that the same principle would apply to his notion of a gravitational force stating that, for any pair of objects, each object in the pair exerts a gravitational attractive force on the other object, the two forces being equal in magnitude though opposite in direction. Thus if a particular object is attracted towards the earth with a specified force, then the earth is attracted towards that object with a force of exactly the same magnitude. We do not ordinarily take the effect on the earth into consideration because the resulting acceleration of the earth is very small, the acceleration of any object by a force of a particular magnitude being inversely proportional to the mass of the accelerated object. In astronomical calculations, where the individual objects are of roughly more comparable mass, both aspects of the gravitational attractions need to be taken into account.

In a person, or in any other animal, all the active supporting forces that can be used to alter the posture of the supported body or to move it around are developed by muscles which are under the control of the central nervous system. "Muscle" and its control can also be a source of confusion. A "muscle" is so called because its activity can appear to feel to the touch like a little mouse moving under the skin (Latin *mus* = mouse, diminutive: *musculus*). But what can be felt in this way is only one of several kinds of contractile tissue in the body. It is distinguishable from the others by two features: 1) suitable histological preparation reveals characteristic cross-banding of the individual cells, and 2) each cell is served by a single nerve fibre connecting it to the central nervous system. Such muscle is spoken of as "striped" or "voluntary," which expresses the property that each cell is made active, in the normal course of events, only by activity in its own special motor nerve fibre. Although each individual striped muscle cell receives its own individual nerve fibre, an individual motor nerve cell, or motoneuron, is connected to several, sometimes several hundred, muscle cells. Since all of these muscle cells will be made active simultaneously when the motoneuron is active, the effective control has to be organised on the basis of the activation of motoneurons, rather than of individual muscle cells or of named muscle masses. We speak of control by motor units, where each "motor unit" consists of one motoneuron together with all the muscle cells served by its branches. A dissectable mass of muscle tissue given a separate anatomical name, such as the "biceps," contains a large number of motor units which may be activated separately in different combinations to produce different overall patterns of force for different purposes. There is thus a good deal of complicated machinery involved between the decision to make a particular voluntary movement and the actual development of the necessary forces to pull appropriately on the bones of the skeleton. None of the stages in the linking machinery is accessible to conscious experience. What we feel depends on messages from deformation receptors that are affected by the resulting movement. We have no direct knowledge of the neurophysiological command process itself. There is, in fact, a huge gap between the world of personal experience and the world of scientific explanation.

The framework of the body consists of a number of separate bones, linked together by flexible joints, from which all the various soft parts are suspended. Because of the joints, the skeleton cannot stand up by itself. The posture of a living animal depends on the activity of muscles. These are arranged in such a way that each is attached, at its ends, to two different bones. We often think of a muscle as "contracting" when it is active, but this is not the whole story. When a muscle cell is made active, it will do one or more of three things: It will shorten if it can; it will develop a tension against a resistance; it will show an increased resistance to extension.

Individual named muscle masses may be distinguished as "extensors" or "flexors" according to whether their activity produces an increase or a decrease in the angle at the joints between the bones to which the muscle is attached. Muscles can only pull, they cannot push, while a bone can push, pull, or act as a lever. The forces exerted by the body against other objects, including the ground, depend on the musculo-skeletal system behaving as a complex triangulated lattice structure, where each triangle consists either of two struts and a tie, or of two ties and a strut, a "tie" being a member in tension and a "strut" being a member capable of supporting a compressive thrust. Such a lattice can transmit forces from one place in the body to another, and can also transform the tensions developed by muscles into thrusts against objects in the environment.

When we reach up to pull down the branch of a tree, what we are actually doing is transferring to the branch some of the support force normally exerted by the feet against the ground. If the branch is robust enough, it can be made to "bear the whole of our weight." That is to say, the arms develop the whole of the stress force needed to provide for the whole body an equal upward acceleration to the downward acceleration attributable to gravity. In the absence of an overhead branch, or something serving the same function, it is not immediately clear to the uninitiated what an Alexander teacher means by the expression "pulling down." It is a jargon expression.

Much of the activity of voluntary muscle, such as in the maintenance of the upright posture and the performance of acts of locomotion, is called forth and coordinated without any awareness of what is going on, so long as everything proceeds smoothly and without unexpected interference. The use of the name "voluntary" for the muscles does not necessarily imply the intervention of the will. The co-ordination of motor activity is achieved unconsciously, using sensory information from many sources. The receptors in muscles, tendons, and joints, along with receptors of a different kind in the inner ear, are grouped together under the name of the "proprioceptive system," to indicate that the relevant receptors are sensitive to changes occurring within the body. Other important contributions come from touch, vision, and hearing.

Actions that are carried out without conscious awareness can be classified under two distinct heads, namely reflex and habitual. In reflex action, both the detection of the "adequate stimulus" and the formulation of the stereotyped response, are dependent on patterns of connection between neurons that are laid down in the developing embryo according to inherited rules. Habits, on the other hand, are patterns of learned behaviour, unrestricted in variety, where the responses have been rehearsed so often that the occurrence of the "trigger gestalt" no longer attracts attention. A "gestalt" is a pattern that can be identified even when some of its constituents are missing. The whole of the background of our perceptual world is constructed from components that are recognised in this way, sometimes even mistakenly, without our paying any particular attention to them. It appears that we can, in fact, direct our attention at a particular time to only a very restricted portion of our total sensory experience at that time, and we usually don't pay attention, either, to the details of our motor activity. Many postural adjustments and components of locomotor acts turn out to be both habitual and unconscious.

It is the variety of the patterns of habitual behaviour adopted by different individuals, together with the great regularity of the patterns seen in a particular individual, that makes it possible for us to recognise certain individuals by their posture and gait. The fact that the trigger for habitual behaviour is detected without attracting attention makes it particularly difficult to change a person's habits. Once the habitual action has been initiated, it usually proceeds to its conclusion without the person being able to do anything about it. The action is performed "without thinking." Many of the problems that lead people to seek the help of Alexander teachers arise from inappropriate postural habits. The amount of muscular effort needed to support the body is at a minimum in a "well-balanced" posture. Departures from this "ideal" call for extra effort and one may be tempted to apply even more effort to provide additional security by activating flexors and extensors simultaneously, thus stiffening certain joints. This extra effort gradually becomes habitual, and it can be quite difficult to break these unhelpful habits.

To have any hope of changing a particular person's habit there are two conditions that must be satisfied. In the first place, the person has to have a strong and genuine desire to change. In some cases where the trigger contains an element of chemical addiction, the helper may need some effort and skill to maintain the necessary motivation. If the motivation is present, the next requirement is that the person has, somehow, to be brought to a condition in which he can become aware of the developing situation in which the habit is likely to be initiated. Here again some skill is called for on the part of the helper, who has to devise ways of directing the client's attention.

The sensations aroused in the client by contact with the teacher's hands encourage the client to make subtle changes to his posture, while at the same time drawing the client's attention to the proprioceptive messages generated at different stages in the lesson. This focussed and heightened attention eventually picks up the condition in which the undesired habits are likely to be initiated, enabling the client to develop that, "Hey, wait a bit!" reaction which provides the opportunity for change. He can then refrain from initiating his formerly habitual response to the situation, giving him the chance to develop an alternative strategy. In the talks printed here, Walter Carrington uses his gentle, almost hypnotic, quiet rhetoric to lead aspiring teachers to learn how to cultivate the appropriate mind-set in their clients so as to enable them to acquire those new postural habits that will so much increase their feeling of well-being.

TRIS ROBERTS
Fintry, Scotland

Author's preface

FOR ALL OF US, to live life to the full would seem a reasonable ambition, but as Alexander pointed out, we cannot hope to fulfil it without a knowledge of what he called the *means whereby*.

His life's work was the demonstration of this means whereby it is possible to translate wishes into actions, and as he claimed, it was the outcome of his experience and observation alone. For him, theoretical speculation played no part. His is a practical Technique, and it has stood the test of time.

When we read his writings, we realise that he was always seeking the best way to explain to us how it had all seemed to him. To understand what he has written we need to have some experience similar to his own. This is not easy to gain, but as we struggle to follow his instructions and, by means of *inhibition* and *direction*, to practice his Technique, his writings become clearer.

These talks, given to the students in our training course for teachers, are some of my attempts to explain his writings in the light of experience gained in my own teaching and also some of the theoretical knowledge that is available today. But as the Chinese proverb says, "it is only the lesson learnt that is of any value," and no theory could justify a practical technique that failed the test of "operational verification." Yet it is interesting to note that nothing has emerged so far of either a practical or theoretical nature to cast doubts on the validity of Alexander's findings. Like him, we must always put practice before theory and always be prepared to test our conclusions by practical results, for as Professor George Coghill expressed it, we are not concerned with Life, but with Living, not with Being but with Becoming and that, for all of us, must be our supreme experiment.

WALTER CARRINGTON
London, England

Editor's note

WALTER CARRINGTON has been training teachers of the Alexander Technique for over 50 years. During much of that time, talks like the ones included in the pages that follow have been an integral part of the training process. His audience during these informal talks has been teachers in training, recent graduates doing a post-graduate term, and his teaching colleagues, some of whom he trained decades earlier.

Literally thousands of times over the years, Walter Carrington has picked up one of F.M. Alexander's four books and has started to read aloud. Sometimes the half hour passes with Mr. Carrington almost exclusively reading, pausing only occasionally to clarify a section of the text. Often, however, he takes a sentence, or a phrase, or sometimes a single word of Alexander's, puts the book down in his lap, with the page marked by a finger, and starts to amplify the meaning of the section that has caught his attention that day. Those are the kinds of talks from which the 29 essays that follow have been selected.

The talks cover a wide range of subjects so that the reader can get a chance to "hear" Walter Carrington's views on giving directions, inhibition, lying down, chair work, positions of mechanical advantage, etc. The main criterion for choosing these particular talks—out of the 150 talks that were considered—was personal and idiosyncratic in nature. I selected those talks that most affected the way I thought about my own use.

These informal spoken essays have continued to influence my teaching and my daily life over the two year span I've been working on this project. That is only fitting since, as Walter Carrington states, the Alexander Technique is a practical technique. And one of the main reasons, perhaps the only reason, these talks have been such an important part of his teacher training program for all these years is that they are practical and relevant to the everyday challenges of teaching and living.

The title for *The Act of Living* came out of one essay in particular, but the idea contained within the title runs throughout the book. Consistent as Walter Carrington's call is for doing less, for making less muscular tension in the acts of life, also consistent throughout this collection is his reminder that life is an act, and that the point of life, as he says in his preface, is to live life fully. The Alexander Technique has no value, no life, as a thing in and of itself. Its value is realized when applied to the world around us. *The Act of Living's* value begins when the ideas in these talks leave the pages of this book and enter the reader's life.

I thank the following people for helping to bring this

project to fruition: For help with the tapes and transcripts: Ginger Beringer, John Brown, Sally Burnay, Jean Fischer, Beryl McLachlan, Daryl Schilling, Beryl Tollady, Miriam Wohl, and, especially, Stephanie Walsh. For giving graciously of their time and words for the preface and introduction: Dr. Tristan Roberts and Glynn Macdonald. Sincere thanks also to book designer Marianne Ackerman, and to Edward and Linda Avak, Galen Cranz, Michael Gelb, Brian McCullough, Jeremy Paul, and Pendragon Press. Thanks to Lorelei, Samuel and Elazar Sontag for bringing joy into every project by Mornum Time Press. And, finally, to Walter Carrington, a special thanks for giving permission to pursue this project, and for the support, friendship and help given over the past seven years.

JERRY SONTAG
San Francisco, California

Introduction

WALTER HADRIAN Marshall Carrington was born in London on May 4th 1915. His father, the Reverend Walter Marshall Carrington was vicar of St. Saviour's, Shepherds Bush. Walter was a chorister at All Saints Church Margaret Street in London and then went to St. Paul's School. Surrounded by music and the spoken word from an early age, Walter developed a great love and understanding of both. He decided to join the order of the Jesuits but changed his plans after his introduction to the Technique through his form master at St. Pauls. He had been given *Man's Supreme Inheritance* to read in the hope that the Technique would be of help to his mother, Hannah Carrington, who was seriously ill and bedridden at the time. Her course of lessons with Alexander enabled her to make a full recovery. Walter's lessons convinced him to join the Training Course for Teachers. After qualifying in 1939 he continued to work on the training course with Alexander as well as give private lessons. When Alexander was no longer able to come in every day for the training course, he asked Walter to take over the day to day running of the course. After Alexander died in 1955, Walter continued teaching and running the Training Course. In

1960 he and his wife Dilys moved to 18 Lansdowne Road in Holland Park and began the Constructive Teaching Centre. It is in the ground floor of this house that Walter gives the morning talks at 12 noon each weekday.

I was introduced to Walter Carrington by my teacher Peggy Williams in 1972. The first thing that I noticed about him was his voice—it literally embodied the Technique for me. I had been told by my singing teacher that I would benefit from Alexander lessons. Not only did I benefit but I felt compelled to join the Training Course. In those days our teachers included Dilys Carrington, Peggy Williams, Winifred Dusseck, Tony Spawforth, Sidney Holland, Mary Holland, Irene Tasker and Ursula Benn. Frank Pierce Jones and Joan and Alex Murray would drop in from America.

The connection between the whole person and the sounds that are being made is known as vocal quality. The listener recognizes a person through the sounds they make. This quality is present in all areas: breathing, vocalization, articulation, thought behind the sound, the meaning behind the words. Walter's vocal quality is unique and extraordinary. His voice has a rich resonance that rings like the bells in old churches. Outside in the hall of 18 Lansdowne Road, we can hear his voice sonorously humming, roundly rising and falling, until it is broken by a great rippling laugh. Voice teachers would describe this sound as coming from a released diaphragm with excellent muscular tone. His laugh has a Rabelaisian quality. The first requirement of the Whispered 'ah' is to be able to think of something funny and this is never difficult when we are with Walter. He is a constant reminder that joy is an important ingredient in our work.

In this second collection of talks, we are given the opportunity to read some of Walter's thoughts. Although we cannot hear his words we are changed by listening to them in our minds. Walter has the rare gift of being able to convey his understanding of the work not only through the words he chooses, but in the very way that he speaks. Such is his vocal skill that when he speaks of 'F.M' or 'Egypt' or 'an old pupil of mine,' as well as hearing the words, we can almost see and feel them.

> *When he speaks, the air, a charter'd libertine is still, and*
> *the mute wonder lurketh in men's ears*
> *To steal his sweet and honey'd sentences*

Over the years his mute hands daily verify the work. When he speaks we are allowed to hear his thoughts and appreciate his deep understanding. Carlyle said that 'language is the garment of our thoughts.' In Walter's case this is a rich tapestry and we are fortunate that this collection of Walter's thoughts has been made available. Sometimes Walter's words can seem surprisingly simple but in this simplicity we can begin to experience the deep meaning, significance and joy of our work.

GLYNN MACDONALD
London, England

Thinking to do

WHEN PEOPLE ARE ASKED to do something, and they go to do it, almost invariably their immediate reaction is to tense up. That's the problem. It is what puts people's reactions so wrong in so many cases. It is absolutely habitual. They tense in response to things, particularly if it's something unfamiliar or unusual or emotionally charged—particularly emotionally charged. Now if you can make a conscious, voluntary habit of responding by inhibiting or, if you like, saying I have time—it doesn't matter how you express the thought to yourself so long as that's what you convey—you've got the time to choose and decide how you're going to carry on from there. That gets you on to a different footing, a different basis altogether. And that is the essence of inhibition. It's not a question, as people very often think, of, "I'm not going to get up out of this chair and wild horses won't drag me." It's not like that. The essential thing about inhibition is the realization that you have the time, you have the possibility, to choose and decide.

In my experience in connection with inhibition in particular and use and function in general, both of myself and of other people, there is so much that goes on at a subconscious level. I don't mean just in the ordinary psychoanalytic sense, in the sense of the ordinary way in which the unconscious is spoken about and so on in psychological terms, but I mean there is such a lot of work in process in the whole neuromuscular system. Nerves are passing messages, both motor messages to muscle and sensory messages from sense organs to the brain. There's all the flow of nervous activity, the flow of muscular activity, there's a tremendous lot going on. When we are doing nothing, when we are not aware that we're doing anything, there's yet a tremendous lot going on and most of it is going on at a level, as we know, far, far below the level of consciousness. And it's important to realize that and acknowledge it, because, at the point when something comes to consciousness, and you have then the possibility of evaluating it, it is so important what happens next.

I'm thinking of a situation that's familiar to everybody here, to anybody who has had an Alexander lesson; that is to say, you're sitting in the chair and the teacher says, now stand up. And so, there's the stimulus, and as a good Alexander pupil you obediently respond to it by saying "no." You then give your orders in response to that cue. But the "no" that you said, now the whole question is: Did you really mean no? What did you mean when you said no? Did you really abandon and reject any thought or intent to stand up, because that's what you're supposed to do, or did you really just say, "I'm not going to stand up now, but I'm going to stand up in a moment?" Did you think, "Well, I'm just saying no and giving the orders as part of the process of going on to stand up." In other words, the objective, the end of standing up, wasn't really inhibited at all. All you did was postpone. Of course, that doesn't achieve the result at all because all the habitual preparation has gone on to quite an advanced point and nothing has really been significantly changed.

So, as you know, in our work, in teaching, it is absolutely critical that you do manage to get people to say no. And to say no in the proper way, because if you're not careful, you'll find that they will say no by adding "wild horses won't make me." And so they say no all right, but they absolutely stiffen every muscle in their bodies.

You've got to get people to an understanding of what is required in response to an act, but you've got to take them further than the understanding. Just the understanding isn't sufficient. It's important on the way to understand, but beyond understanding, they've jolly well got to wish it, they've got to want it, they've got to have the real desire or wish to proceed in that particular way. So, in a sense, inhibition is very simple and should be quite an easy matter. The difficulties that we make about it are very likely of our own making.

In working with small children, we used to make inhibition a game, and it was a game that the children usually enjoyed very much and got the point of very well because the experience of life of most small children is that they're not supposed to inhibit. They're supposed to hurry up and get on with it and do what they're told and wake up and think what they're doing and all the rest of it. They're not supposed to hang about and when asked to do something, say "No, I shan't." It's considered to be quite out of order. So when you say, as we used to say to them, "Now I'm going to ask you to do something and instead of doing it I want you to say, no I shan't," they think that's perfectly hilarious. And of course, as they gained more experience they realized that what it really meant was that saying no gave them more independence and freedom of choice, that they weren't just being dragged along helter skelter.

A little story that just occurred to me was that as it came towards Christmas at the Little School—which was located at 16 Ashley Place, Alexander's Teaching Rooms, and was started by his assistant, Irene Tasker, in 1924—it was thought that there ought to be a Christmas party, that everybody ought to get together and put on a big do, some sort of a do for Christmas. And so the nature of this do was being discussed, people were making various suggestions, but one of the children piped up and said, "No. We can't possibly have a do, that would be quite wrong. What we must have is a non-do." So the Christmas party came to be called the non-do.

Now mostly, in life, you're thinking to do, you're thinking to act, because life is an act, not a thought. And if you keep in mind that all the pathways in the brain lead directly or indirectly to muscle, as indeed they do, you can see that what is happening in your brain, what you're thinking, is going to have an effect on muscle. So here you are, thinking thoughts that are, so to speak, twitching your muscles. What you've got to realize is that it is also possible to think thoughts which don't twitch your muscles, that actually cause your muscles to be left alone and not excited and not stimulated. And that is the process of inhibitory thinking that we call leaving yourself alone. That is the state or process that we are trying to bring about in our pupils when we give them an Alexander lesson. When that happens, when that thought process begins, we can begin to get the works to work.

General functioning

As I've often pointed out, it is very important to keep reminding ourselves that in science, in the general way of things, there isn't any concept of general functioning. As Alexander teachers, we have a concept of general functioning because we are well aware of how our manner of use affects our general functioning. If you pull down then it inevitably affects your breathing, circulation, digestion and everything else. It is perfectly possible to pull down in such a way that perhaps you do more damage to your circulation than you do to your breathing. Or you can pull down in such a way that you really do terrible damage to your breathing but happen to be endowed with a cast iron stomach. You can get all these variations, but the fact of the matter is if you pull down your general functioning will be adversely affected.

On the other hand, if you can manage to get some direction going and get yourself going up a bit, that will raise the standard of general functioning. The same line of reasoning applies, however; that's to say, when you start going up you know that it will be beneficial but you've got to see how it's going to be beneficial. Your perception of your problem may be that you've got rotten digestion or rotten circulation. You start to go up and it may well appear that everything else improves except the circulation or digestion or whatever it was that you were looking at.

Pain is a good example of this principle. It can most certainly happen that people come for lessons because they have pain that troubles them and they can have lessons and their general functioning is improved enormously and their friends see them moving differently and say, "You look so different, what have you been doing?" Still, the pain persists. So you can't guarantee that as you raise the standard of general functioning that it will produce the specific change that you are looking for. And, equally, you can't be certain that if you depress the standard of general functioning that it will necessarily produce the adverse affect that you would expect that it would straight away. People with very bad use can very often get away with all sorts of things, but then you've got to remember life is very unfair and there is no justice. That is what you have to bear in mind.

When we talk of the manner of use, we are apt to fall into the habitual trap of separation. We may find ourselves thinking in physical terms, in terms of body tissue, muscles, bones and all that sort of thing, perhaps nerves too. But we exclude thoughts and feelings and wishes and emotions and all the mental side of the thing. Manner of use is a holistic concept that not only includes the

thoughts and feelings and emotions, but also, of para-
mount consideration, includes your desire and your
will. That is the primary consideration. It always boils
down in the end to what you want and finding out
what you want.

When you want something, your body proceeds to set
about working in accordance with what you want. Of
course when you are confronted with a situation where
there is evident misuse, you can say nobody really wants
misuse. And, of course, you'd be right. No one wants
misuse, but they can be so confused and muddled in their
wants that the confused signals, the confused messages,
activate the musculature in such a way that misuse is the
invariable result.

So if you are able to exercise inhibition so that you
identify what you don't want to happen and jolly well
see that it doesn't happen, you can make change in your
use so that your general functioning will improve. But
for that to happen, it does come back, in the end, to the
question of the will.

Habits of thought and action

THE MOST COMMON, the most critical, habit of thought and action is the habit of approaching any task by making an increase in muscular effort—in other words, tensing or stiffening in order to respond. That habit of tensing and tightening is pretty well universal and one of the commonest difficulties that you encounter in trying to teach this technique.

If you got together a whole lot of coaches and experts from all kinds of different disciplines, whether it's sport or the arts or so on, they will confirm that the greatest difficulty you have at the outset is to prevent people from this response of increased tension. This reaction has the effect of making learning and communication extremely difficult. As soon as somebody has tensed up to do something, they're usually not in the proper frame of mind to take in what you're trying to say to them. Choose any form of instruction you'd like—the tennis coach, the golf instructor, the voice teacher—the moment you give people the stimulus to do some-thing, they respond by tensing up. In doing so the pupil has very largely prevented any understanding, any appreciation, of what is required to be successful at that activity.

That is the first habit that you are up against. But the problem goes deeper than that. Not only is the original reaction of increased tension a large problem, but then there is the very, very quick assessment of what is to be done, an assessment made with little thought and little observation of the situation. It would be a big step if you could get people not to start with the increased tension, and then to go on and actually appraise the whole situation and see what is to be done. So when they actually come to carry the whole process out, they do so by watching all the time, not merely whether they're being successful in the narrow sense of the task that they've set themselves, but what the incidental consequences are that they hadn't foreseen or hadn't expected. When you're doing anything in life, the more aware you can be of not only the process but also the consequences, the more it's possible to change and modify the carrying out of the process itself. And of course one particular direction in which you always seek to modify is towards economy of effort. Quite clearly there is no sense in carrying something out, whether it be a new task or one you've faced many times before, by doing it in such a way that you're making a whole lot more effort than is actually necessary.

To get people to make that sort of change in their habit and in their outlook and in their performance requires going beyond just appealing to their reason. It is a psychophysical change that is really necessary. It isn't just habits of thought, it's habits of action. It's the entire habitual setup within the organism that is going to have to be modified if you're going to make a successful change. And that is what our teaching is really all about.

When you are setting out to give somebody an Alexander lesson, you are trying to deal with exactly this sort of problem. That is why, first of all, you're trying to calm them down so they have a chance to withhold the immediate response and to reduce the level of strain and tension. With that change, the general functioning of the body can work with less interference because it's only when other aspects of general functioning, like breathing and circulation and digestion and particularly the postural mechanism, are working at a reasonably satisfactory level can you expect the brain to begin to operate. You can't possibly get the little gray cells to operate if you are holding your breath and pulling down and interfering with all the works. So it is a total process of change and it's change that goes against habit.

Habit is the thing that gets in the way of change. If people's habitual reaction is a fear reaction, which in many cases it is, you really have got difficulties. It's bad enough to change habits where people are only clinging to a rather nice feeling or a nice comfortable sensation. As an old pupil of mine once said, "A groove is a very comfortable thing." That's bad enough, but if you're actually afraid of being drawn out of the groove, if you're afraid of what may happen if you get out of it, then that makes it even more difficult. Then you really have got a challenge in front of you.

Sciatica

AS MOST PEOPLE KNOW, sciatica is inflammation of the sciatic nerve. The sciatic nerves are very large nerves that come out in the lower part of the spine and go down the legs. When those nerves are annoyed and pressed and damaged, you get a very nasty pain down the legs. It is generally recognized that sciatic pain is brought about by accidents and pressures and stresses that press on the nerve. If you recall your anatomy and just think of the base, the lower part of the spine where you have the sacrum, and the bits that are fused together to form the spade shaped structure that slots into the pelvis, then where this spade shaped structure slots in you've got a very, very strong joint binding the connection between the spine and the pelvic bones.

Now I can remember years ago when I was still training, and even afterwards when I was teaching, the accepted wisdom of the orthopedic surgeons was that those sacroiliac joints, as they are called, are so strong that movement there is really quite out of the question. So when osteopaths and other quacks and unqualified people claimed that sciatica was caused by damage or displacement of the sacro-iliac joint, the orthopedic people said nonsense. They said rubbish, it can't happen. But of course nowadays the outlook has changed considerably and people have been forced to acknowledge that the osteopaths were perfectly right, and that there is quite a lot of potential movement in the sacro-iliac joints in some people, and some people do manage therefore to twist and distort themselves in ways that cause sciatica.

So I'm just mentioning all that as being quite interesting, that in a fairly short time outlook and opinion have changed from those days when osteopathy was pretty well a dirty word as far as orthodox medicine was concerned, to now when you've got quite a number of doctors who have done courses in osteopathy.

But coming back to our work, the question to address is can or does the Alexander technique cure sciatica? And the answer to that is, no. It does not. It doesn't and indeed can't cure anything in that way. But if you can change somebody's manner of use so that instead of pulling themselves down, they generate a little bit of upward energy, free themselves and move in a better manner, then that does relieve a lot of the tension and the stress. In so doing, you contribute very significantly to an improvement in the condition.

In saying this, we're not just pussyfooting around. What we're really emphasizing is that, whereas if somebody's got sciatica and they go to the doctor and they get some anti-inflammatory drug administered one way or the other, the chances are that at least temporarily you can reasonably expect to ease the pain. With lessons in the Alexander Technique, it will be a very individual matter, and how quickly or how long it will take before there is any change in the pain situation will depend very much on individual circumstances. From a practical point of view, if somebody comes along with sciatica and they have lessons expecting they're going to be cured of sciatica and they're going to get instant relief, they may be very, very disappointed indeed. Whereas if it can be made clear to them that what they are going to do is to change their manner of reaction and change their relative functioning, and if they really do pay attention to that then they will benefit enormously, far beyond just the relief of the sciatic symptoms—which almost certainly will come about eventually, but nobody can safely predict when. So it is quite important to make these distinctions clear because they really reflect the fundamental character of our work. It will help pupils understand what we are attempting to do, and what we are not attempting to do.

SEPTEMBER 22, 1989

What you don't want

IN OUR WORK AND TEACHING, we use
words like "direction" and "order" and even "thinking,"
but quite simply the essence of the matter is what you
want—and, even more important, what you don't want.
If you really and truly don't want something, then it is the
preventive messages, the preventive activity in the brain,
that are necessary to insure that what you want to have
stopped is stopped. When those preventive messages are
sent, there's no way in which you're going to find yourself doing what you don't want to do and don't intend to
do. That is the crux of the matter.

It's our common experience of life that we go and do
things and then we say, "Oh, I didn't mean to do that, I
didn't mean to do it like that, I didn't mean to do that at
all." We get into such a muddle, and at the core of the
muddle is that we haven't made up our blessed minds. We
haven't really been clear in our minds what we want and
what we don't want. So if you half want something and
half want something else, there's endless confusion.

To give a concrete example, you are sitting in a chair,
and in the depths of your subconscious the wish is being

expressed that you should stand up. All the nerve messages are being sent to bring about the habitual pattern, the habitual manner of use for standing up in the habitual way. The whole familiar pattern of activity is activated. In the ordinary teaching situation where you're sitting in a chair and about to stand up, if the teacher asks you to stand up and he's going to leave it to you actually to stand up, it's pretty certain that you will set about doing it in a way that feels right. That is to say you will do what you feel is necessary to be done in order to stand up. So, for example, in order to stand up you may feel that what you need to do is to lean forward. You can justify this by saying, "Well I need to get the weight more over my feet before I straighten my legs." But the fact of the matter is that whatever justification you put forward, you feel that the thing to do is to lean forward. And if you feel that that's what you've got to do to get up, well that's what you will do. If somebody says "No, you shouldn't lean forward, what you should do is lean back," then that feels quite wrong and you will soon find lots of reasons that you can put forward to try and argue that it is wrong.

So what is needed is somebody's got to come along, they've got to put their hands on you, and they've got to introduce you to a different experience. It feels quite unfamiliar at first, but then as it's repeated, then it begins to feel more possible. Then it does begin to feel a bit right, and then, as it goes on, it begins to feel a bit more right. It certainly ceases to be unfamiliar and unknown and you're now getting experience of a new, different way. That's what happens to us all. Provided we take the time and the trouble, the new different way becomes a possibility and a reality and something that you can manage.

But of course, you won't manage it if you're fussed and in a hurry and anxious and upset, because when it's a quick and thoughtless reaction, you go back to the old familiar thing, to the old thing that still feels right in your heart of hearts. To have a chance to make a change, you must pause and give yourself time.

You can have lots of lessons and you can get the new way feeling familiar, and you're able to carry out the new way successfully if you give yourself a little time and you stop and think, but the old reflex patterns are still there. So, if you really want to be safe, if you really do want to make the change, you have to go beyond just having lessons and getting the new experience, you've got to think about it. You've got to use your mind. You've got to not only experience, but you've got to make an attempt to understand the significance of the experience. You've got to explain the experience to yourself. It calls for a lot of mental work.

One of the familiar things that people say when they're having Alexander lessons is, "If I won the pools, I'd have a lesson from you every day." Well, that may sound nice, but what they mean is that having the repetition of the experience is lovely, but they haven't got any plans at all to try and understand or use any brain or intelligence or any mental process connected with it. They are just content to leave it at the level of the changed experience during the lesson, and really that is no good.

Now, of course, if you are saying, "Well, yes, I am going to try and understand this, I really am going to try and help myself. I really will try and put this into practice," then a word of caution, a word of warning. Remember, if you're going to succeed, you will have to take it quietly and gently, and keep very calm and take lots of time and you've got to be fairly easy on yourself, you've got to get yourself in a calm frame of mind, a calm attitude, and you've got to stay that way. That's what it is about.

Taking the pressure off

IN OUR WORK, WE WANT to go up in such a way that we take pressure off the joints. If we are going into monkey or going to sit down in a chair, we let our knees go in such a way that we take pressure off the joints, so that the joints work more freely. Now if you then pause and ask yourself, "How is that possible? With my knowledge of physiology and anatomy, how is it conceivable that I can really take the pressure off my knees when I know perfectly well that the weight of all the rest of my body is being taken through my knees as it is transmitted through the feet to the floor?" You might find yourself very puzzled by thinking how can all that happen.

But just for a moment switch the whole thought round and think, "Now if I make myself heavy, if I pull myself down, if I stiffen, it is perfectly evident that my knees don't bend freely." The weight is still the same; of course it is the same. But you can try it and it is something that the experience will make absolutely clear. If you make yourself heavy and pulled down, you will very quickly find that your knees don't work freely. So you then don't stop and say, "I wonder why that is? I wonder why that is so?" What you do is recognize that it is a very wrong and harmful thing to do and you take good care not to do it.

The point that I am just trying to make is that the thing of practical importance to recognize is that I mustn't pull myself down. I mustn't stiffen and tighten when I am going to sit or going into monkey because it puts pressure on all the joints. It puts the whole thing wrong. It is of practical importance to recognize because then you can do your best to see that you don't do it; whereas, if you start speculating about the mechanism and saying, "I wonder how on earth it is possible to be more light and to be more free? How can I take pressure off the joints?" you don't know and you are not likely to find out in any short space of time. It certainly won't contribute at all to the essential task of being observant and alert not to tighten and stiffen and pull down. In fact, while you are pondering all these problems and difficulties you may well be pulling yourself down to do it, because when people get into that sort of mode of thinking they tend to go down rather than to go up.

So, leaving the theoretical behind, on a practical note, here you are lying down on the table with your knees bent. You are directing the knees up to the ceiling because you want, so far as you can, to promote the lengthening of the thigh muscles. In particular, what you want to ensure is that the thigh muscles are not shortening and tightening. While you are on the table, if you go and lift the foot without thought and direction, you will undoubtedly use the muscles in such a way that there will be an awful lot of shortening and contraction and the movement will be relatively stiff. Whereas if you put in the appropriate direction to start with and secure the length, then you will find that the actual lifting of the foot falls into place in the context of the whole activity and works lightly and freely. But this is something that you really have to learn from experience. You try it out and it is open to anybody to make the experiment and see whether it works for them or not. It isn't a theoretical matter. This is a practical affair. It is something to try out.

So again here you are lying on the table with your knees bent and you are going to bring up a foot. Well if you don't immediately pause and say no, you will have already set in motion all the preparation for lifting up the foot in the habitual way. What you have got to do is leave the foot where it is, not try to move it, not to think of moving the foot. But you have got to pay attention to the leg, to the thigh, to the knee and you have got to be thinking of the knee going up to the ceiling. So that as you lie there it is as though your hands were otherwise occupied and somebody was saying to you, "Where is the ceiling?" and with your knee you said, "It's up there." That is the direction that you give with the knee to allow the foot to work freely.

It is absolutely critical for the foot to work properly.

There are lots of muscles in the foot, and of course the foot has to support all the weight of the body and take all the stress and pressure and shock of walking. People tighten and contract the feet and you get two extremes. You get the fallen arch and flat foot or you get the very contracted, bunched up foot with a very high arch. Both conditions are really pretty disastrous.

The foot is supposed to be a tripod with the three weight bearing points—heel, outer margin behind the little toe, and the head of the metatarsal bone at the base of the big toe. The foot needs to be very mobile and free with all the muscles concerned in good working order and lengthening. The joints are not being compacted and compressed but they are being maintained in a state of freedom as much as possible. Well then, what happens when you have got a free foot like that? You could say that the more you go up, the more lengthening you get right through from the foot as the head leads the way to the ceiling. As you lengthen in this manner, the foot will be gathered up a little. You don't want to say contracted. It isn't contracted in a bad sense, but it is just gathered up so that you are standing very lightly and efficiently on the foot. The more freely you go up, the better the foot makes contact with the floor.

Just one more thing that I should add while we are about it is that there is a very close relationship between what happens with your feet and your breathing and use of voice and so on for a very simple practical reason. The only efficient way to sing and use your voice is to go up, and the more you want to use your voice, the more sound you want to produce, the larger the voice, the more you have got to go up to do it. And of course going up is going up. It involves the whole of you—it involves the feet, it involves the legs, it involves it all.

The feet

THE FOOT IS MADE UP of quite a collection of bones that are held together by the whole complex of muscles that effectively pull the bones together like springs. The function of these muscles is to bind the bones together, to collect them all together and ensure that they form the longitudinal arch and the transverse arch of the foot. The arch is necessary because it provides for shock absorbing so that when the weight has gone to the foot, you've got a spring there to absorb the shock.

The way in which these bones are collected together form into the arched structure which involves the muscles of the leg and the thigh. The simple thing to remember is that the muscles of the leg and the thigh work in a spiral. When the leg is bent, the knee and the whole structure spirals outwards; when the leg is straightened, it spirals inward.

The pulls that are involved in that spiral process keep the bones of the foot together in such a manner that the whole foot is spring-loaded. When the pulls are working properly, the arches are established and sustained. As long as you've got that free working in the long muscles that control the whole leg, then the arch will be fine.

If you get interference with this free spiral pull of the muscles, then you get fixation and rigidity. Fixation and rigidity as far as the foot is concerned usually means a very high arch. It means the whole foot becomes compressed and bunched up and contracted. The other extreme is when the pulls don't work and the whole thing collapses. There's nothing to draw the bones together, and then as the weight comes onto it, the whole structure spreads and then you've got the flat foot, which is painful and disastrous.

But one critical thing to keep in mind when thinking about the foot and the formation of the arch is that the creation and sustaining of the arch doesn't stop at the musculature of the thigh. It doesn't stop at the pelvis. It doesn't stop in the lower back. It's the whole of the body's musculature right the way through that is working in a way that generates an upthrust. When you get that overall lengthening, so that the whole tendency is upwards, then you've got the muscle tone, you've got the condition that draws the bones together in the proper way. You've got the arches. You've got the spring. Then you've got what you want.

But the effect of the whole system on the foot is something that is almost totally disregarded in physiotherapy, and in chiropody and things like that. People dealing with the feet realize that flat feet and fallen arches are painful and tiring and badly damaging. One of the most frequent attempts at correcting this problem directly is by prescribing arch supports. You wear an arch support in the shoe, which then holds the arch in place. This arch support does nothing for the whole of the vital force—the upward working of the whole of the neuromuscular system. It doesn't address that at all.

The arch support changes the shape of the arch, but it hasn't done anything about the springing, it hasn't done anything about the shock-absorbing. There's nothing to absorb the shock as you put the foot down on the ground. The arch support relieves tiredness for the time being. It feels a little better than flat feet, but it isn't really getting to the root of the problem.

The other thing that people very often prescribe for flat feet or fallen arches are exercises. They very often advocate that instead of standing so that you have the toes turned out at 45 degrees to each other, very often when people have fallen arches they are recommended to be sure to always have the feet parallel. By insisting on keeping the feet parallel, the pulls on the calf muscles, and on the muscles of the lower leg tend to support the arch. Whereas, if the foot is turned out, and of course the muscles aren't working, then the foot, you might say, collapses and the arch disappears into the foot. Again, like the arch support, the parallel feet may create more of an arch but only at the expense of the legs, the torso, the whole structure itself.

All sorts of remedies are attempted for fallen arches and flat feet and so on, but unless the whole working of what we call the primary control is taken into consideration, then the vital force doesn't flow properly in the arch, and these particular measures won't do anything really about it. You need to get to the root of the problem and the only way in which to get to the root of the problem is by considering how first of all you use the foot, but then of course how you use the whole of yourself. It always comes back to that. You've got to think of it from that point of view. You've got to think of the overall picture of how you use yourself, the total coordination. The other approaches will only give temporary help and people will continue to suffer.

The balance of the head

ON THE JOINT WHERE THE HEAD is articulated on the end of the spine, there is a fairly limited range of movement. According to anatomists, it is a range of movement which we can say quite definitely is under 30 degrees of arc. If you try to move the head further down than 30 degrees, the other joints of the neck get involved and the neck itself comes forward.

With most people who are pulled down and who have really shortened into themselves, they have turned the base of the neck into a major joint so that they tend to move the head and neck together as one unit. They don't think or see much separation between the head and the neck. As a matter of fact, when people really pull the head back, their neck, as you can imagine, gets very much involved and the curve of the neck inevitably is exaggerated. The neck has to curve forward to allow the head to come back to that extent. So we don't want the head to go back at all. And when it comes to the head going forward, we want to allow the head to move to the full extent that the atlanto-occipital joint will permit, which is quite a small amount, and not to exceed that.

Because if you try to put the head any further forward, inevitably it will involve the neck as well, and the neck will start going forward from the joint at the 7th cervical—where the last neck bone sits on the first thoracic bone.

If you get neck involvement in the movement and the poise of the head, then if the head moves, the neck moves with it. This relationship causes tension in the neck muscles. It involves a degree of tension and compression in the neck joints and it is very easy to understand that if you've got that then you are going to disturb the larynx. You are going to compress it or to interfere with it. In other words, you are going to put it wrong. Here is the larynx, this cartilaginous structure that is made of the cartilages that protect the vocal cords and protect the passages. This structure is in place in a complex web of muscles designed, on the one hand, to allow it to move freely and, on the other hand, to ensure that when the rest of the structure of the body moves, then all the force, the stress that is generated in the movement, is damped out by the time it reaches the larynx so that the larynx remains sitting there unaffected by the movement around it. The larynx has got to rise when you swallow. The structure has got to come up so that the epiglottis can work, so that when you are taking food down the food passage, you don't want it to get misdirected and go down the air passage. So it is very important that in swallowing the mechanism should work to close off the air passage so that the food passage is open and fine. But the rest of the time you want the air passage as free as possible so that the whole of the vocal mechanism is able to do its own complex work without interference. But this freedom can not occur if the head goes back or goes too far forward.

So if we can just clear this situation up a little bit further: Let us say that backward and forward on the atlanto-occipital joint describes a very small range of movement. The difference between the head going backwards and forwards on that joint is very small. As soon as you go beyond that shift backwards and forwards, you are no longer balancing. You are adding a downward force to the head, and as soon as you add down to that delicate balance, you are in deep trouble.

You have a very small movement, but within that range of movement it is critical that the head should not go back. It needs to be in forward range so that the tendency is always forward and not back. I know you all know this, but looking at the skeleton, looking at the skull, the way that the mass of the skull is disposed on the joint is such that the weight operates a little in front of the joint. The joint is not under the head as you would have a billiard ball on a billiard cue if you were trying to balance the ball on the cue. The head would not sit on the end of the spine if it were not for the muscles gently restraining it from its natural tendency to fall forward. The tendency to fall forward is natural and absolutely what is supposed to happen all the time. If you tighten the muscles excessively, if you stiffen them, the head gets pulled back and the whole mechanism is interfered with. Serious consequences result throughout the whole organism because that balance of the head is a very important feature in what we call primary control.

If you pull the head hard back, the curve of the neck can really be exaggerated. So the curves of the spine can be increased and decreased. As that happens, you lengthen and shorten in stature. But in addition to that there is the fact that all the joints—hip, knee, ankle joints for instance—are all encapsulated in an arrangement whereby there is quite a bit of play in the joints. You can put pressure on the joints and compress them or you can take pressure off and release them considerably. And although the difference that can be made by compressing the joints and decompressing them may be quite small, it is of practical significance, because if the joints are under pressure they don't work as freely as they do if you take the pressure off. So this contribution to lengthening or shortening in stature is quite important.

The word stature is useful to use because we are taking into consideration all these different factors that contribute to lengthening or shortening. We are not just focusing on one set of factors like the increase or decrease of the curves. This again is more than just of theoretical importance because when you come to think about yourself and think about other people you are looking to avoid shortening in stature. That is obviously what you want to prevent. You want to prevent not only some shortening, you want to prevent any shortening. You don't merely want to prevent the curves of the spine being excessive, you want to prevent the compression on the spinal joints. You want to eliminate anything that contributes to shortening, and promote anything that contributes to lengthening.

You may believe that you don't know sufficient anatomy to list all the things that contribute to shortening or lengthening. Still, your objective, very definitely, is to lengthen in stature. And since you want to lengthen in stature you will be looking about and observing to see anything that will contribute to that, anything that will help, and equally, eliminate anything that will hinder. So the concept of lengthening in stature is a very important one. It is all too easy in physical training, in exercises, in sports and dance and all sorts of different things that people do, to start looking at specific pieces of the puzzle, to look at this bit or that bit, to look at arthritic joints or whatever it may be, and when you start focusing on the bits and pieces, it is very easy to lose the overall view. Our whole technique is very much concerned with the overall view because what we want is lightness and freedom, starting with the head balancing on the neck, yes, and encompassing an overall lengthening in stature.

The length and the width

IN OUR WORK, with all of the focus we place on the head/neck relationship, it is easy to get lulled into thinking that all you need pay attention to is the neck. But Alexander was very clear about this, and I want to be clear as well, that I don't believe that by just paying attention to the neck, and letting the head go forward and up that you are going to correct everything else. That's not how it works. You have to be alive and on the alert to see what is happening all together: to see how you're standing, how your pupil is standing, what is going on in all different areas in order to correct it.

Of course what that means is that you have the pupil standing there in front of you. You get the pupil looking out and not trying to do anything except leaving him or herself alone and inhibiting. Then, with your hands, you take the pupil in such a way that you correct the balance not only of the head but of the whole body. It isn't only the head. It can't only be the head.

You get the pupil into a position of mechanical advantage. Mechanical advantage is a position or a situation, a condition perhaps, in which lengthening of all the different muscles is being promoted so that lengthening of the musculature is taking place, and thereby the springing function of the muscles is being activated. That activation is a necessity before going into action so that you have the proper muscle tone. That proper muscle tone is your mechanical advantage. Because if you haven't got the muscles working properly in turn, then you are laboring under a mechanical disadvantage, and of course that just makes life even more difficult.

So your job, your responsibility, is to bring the pupil into a position of mechanical advantage. The next step is to get the pupil to rehearse the mental orders necessary to sustain the change required. But rehearsing the orders means more than just saying, "neck to be free, head forward and up, back to lengthen and widen." It means actually thinking of freedom of the neck so that we're not stiffening it; actually thinking of the head so that the head is freely poised and is going forward and up and you're really thinking about the back and so on. Not just saying the words, but actually thinking the thoughts. It is above all a matter of thought and observation.

So what this thought process gets for us is the length and the width. And of course just to remember that when we are talking about the widening of the back, what we are particularly thinking of is what is happening with the ribs and shape of the rib cage. People very often forget that the adult rib cage is not a circular structure, it's an elliptical structure—that is to say, the distance from side to side is much greater than the distance from back to front. That's the natural shape of the rib cage.

What we need to do as we secure the length, letting the head go forward and up, and getting the length, we want to insure that the ribs are able to move outwards, sideways, to secure the width. Gaining the width on the long axis of the ellipse sets the condition from which next you can get the maximum depth, i.e. distance between the spine and breastbone. But you have to get widening first—it's getting that opening out that is critical before you try and get the depth. Putting it another way, most people, when they think of expanding the chest, think of throwing the chest out, of raising the chest and throwing it out and moving in front. They think the expansion of the chest is in front, whereas we know that the true expansion of the chest is a matter of getting the width. You have to get the lengthening of the spine first of course so that the pupil is not pulling down; then, on that basis, you go for the widening.

Something that Alexander was always pointing out to us is that when you are working on people you want to watch the process of lengthening and the process of widening. It's very, very easy to get so involved for instance in the lengthening that as you lengthen up you start to narrow without realizing it. Or, alternatively, you see the importance of getting the width and so you work to expand and get the width and you don't realize it at first, but as you widen, you shorten. If you will only remember that when you are working on the widening, keep a watchful eye on the length to see that the length is maintained, or when you're working on the length, keep a watchful eye on the widening to see that the widening is maintained. Alexander said if you do that, if you remember to do that, you've got a built-in check—you can't go wrong, you can't make a mistake, because if you watch one while you're doing the other, it's self-checking. He said, "It's not only fool-proof, it's damned fool-proof." That's what you have to remember.

Coordinated use

THE WHOLE PROCESS OF LEARNING this technique, of having lessons and so on, is to develop coordinated use. But what is coordinated use, you might be asked. It is a very difficult thing to define and describe and put into words.

To put it into words is very, very difficult because it's a whole process of thought and action that is the product of the application of the Technique. We can simplify our description by saying that it is the proper use of the primary control. That can mean something to us, but it doesn't mean anything to people who haven't had similar experiences to our own. What you need to point out, what you need to remember, is that coordinated use involves balance, poise, the mechanical requirements of coping with gravitation. The demands that arise from the circumstances, from the effect of gravity, from the effect of the weight on the different parts of the body, are all satisfactorily met when one's use is coordinated, so that as an outcome you are light, free, mobile, and flexible. With that background of efficient mechanical working throughout the whole organism you are now in position to be able to utilize this working for the given end, the task at hand.

It means that you have, with knowledge and experience and everything, ensured that you've brought about an efficient working of the complex machinery of ourselves. And once you've established the proper working, the critical issue is whether you have control of it. Control of it is what you need because if you haven't got control of the complex mechanism then you're going to be in awful trouble when you go to undertake some voluntary activity.

If you've got the mechanism in working order, then you've still got to want to use it. This is the thing that we're always coming up against in teaching, in everyday practice, because we say to people, "Look, don't try to do it, you don't have to do it and you mustn't try to do it, but if you don't want it to happen there's absolutely no earthly reason why it should happen, so you've got to want it." Don't do it, but want it. That's the challenge. How you get people to want it is one of the great difficulties. You know, it's the old saying of taking the horse to water and persuading it to drink. Well, if you can induce it to taste, it may like it and that may then stimulate it in fact to drink. But it is very difficult to motivate people to want something. If you can't get them to taste, you can't get them to try. This is a very profound, simple truth that we come up against in our work all the time.

And you see this is where the treatment business comes

in, because people come to have Alexander lessons on a treatment basis and both consciously and subconsciously they are very largely satisfied with their own conditions. Their dissatisfaction is only just in some small direction, or relatively small direction, in which they're seeking your help. They're saying, "Treat this, put this right, and everything will be fine, and it will be fine because then I can go on as before. I know how I want to live, I know all about it, but I've got this pain or this or that which is an impeding factor. Cure that for me, and I'll be fine." The change they are looking for is not global in nature. It is very narrow, very specific. Confronted with that attitude it is very, very difficult to bring about the change, and particularly the motivation to change, that we need and that we're talking about.

Working towards a coordinated use is a very different business from solving this or that specific problem. It is all well and good to be concerned with this pain or that, but we are working towards something more fundamental. It is worthwhile to keep an interest in working toward a coordinated use in the front of your mind. It won't always be in the front of your pupil's mind, but you can help them to start to see the problems in this broader light.

The mechanics of the situation

RIGHT, A LITTLE COURSE in elementary anatomy. I recommend to anybody who hasn't got a simple anatomy textbook of their own to look around and try and get one because it is very valuable. It's very, very important to know something about basic anatomy.

Now we nearly always start anatomy with a look at the skeleton and with the consideration of the bones. But I want to begin with something a bit more preliminary. The fact of the matter is this: It is astonishing that doctors, surgeons, nurses, physiotherapists, physical training teachers, people of all kinds who deal with the human body, ignore and are very largely ignorant about the principles of mechanics. It was Leonardo da Vinci, who said in fifteen hundred and something, that if you want to understand anything about the human body, you've got to understand something about the laws of mechanics. And this is absolutely true. It is astonishing that people don't pay attention to the laws of mechanics. They get themselves into such terrible muddles and difficulties through this simple ignorance.

Here we are on this planet and one of the major

influences in our lives is the force of gravity. Gravity is drawing everything towards the center of the earth and all living things have to have, and do have, some sort of a built-in arrangement that enables them to make use of gravity. Gravity is thought of somehow as an enemy and something to be fought, whereas when you really look into mechanics and look into the reality of things, gravity is one of our best friends. Gravity is a tremendous source of energy and it's a tremendous help in our lives. You don't want to look at gravity in a negative way, you want to look at it as something that is really helpful and useful; then it's up to you to take advantage of it. It's one of God's gifts, if you like. It's marvelous stuff!

We human beings have obviously developed a way of going around on two feet. You might think this makes dealing with gravity a great deal more difficult. You might say that the easiest way to deal with gravity is to lie down on the floor because you're perfectly safe there. Or, if you're a creature with a lot of legs, then gravity is okay too, because you've always got a few legs in contact with the ground, and that's going to keep your balance for you and save you all kinds of trouble.

But we only have two legs, and to make matters more challenging, we usually use them one at a time. People think because we've got two legs that we're using them both together all the time, but we're scarcely ever using two legs together. We're always either standing on one or standing on the other, or about to stand on one or about to stand on the other. We are always moving from one foot to the other, from one leg to the other.

In order to stand on two feet, properly on two feet, you've really got to pause and think what you're doing. The fact of the matter is that we have to find our balance. If we're not going to fall over, if we're going to manage to move around securely, if we're going to be light and free through our body, then we've got to find a way so that the whole neuromuscular mechanism—the nerves and muscles, the bones, why speak of the bits, it's the whole, the whole of you and me—is light and free and mobile.

From a practical point of view, what you have to do is, first of all, find your proper shape, which includes your full height. If you are out of shape, you are complicating the issue. You are distorting yourself and making the problem of balance more difficult. After you find your proper shape, then you find your overall balance. And when you've found your balance, then you are in a situation where the amount of neuromuscular energy needed to support you is reduced to the minimum.

Think for a moment of what happens if you are out of shape and out of balance. You are in danger of falling over. In order not to fall over, you are bound to make a lot more muscular effort. When I say that people, scientists, doctors, all these people, ignore mechanics, they don't look at a patient who comes in to the consulting room and say, "Now, you are expending a tremendous amount of energy to stop yourself from falling over, from falling down, that's what you're doing most of all. If you were in better shape, literally in better shape mechanically, if you were in better balance, then you wouldn't be making all this enormous effort to hold yourself up. If you weren't making all that effort to hold yourself up, then probably your muscles wouldn't be as painful, your joints wouldn't be as stiff and fixed and, above all, there's a chance that you might be able to breathe. Because, while you're making all this effort to stand, that effort is absolutely in conflict with the whole set-up that is needed for free breathing, because all muscular effort tends to lead to thoracic rigidity." Alexander was always quoting and repeating, "All muscular effort tends to promote thoracic rigidity." So whenever you make muscular effort, watch the effect on your breathing.

If you're going to help yourself from a conscious and intelligent point of view, then you need conscious awareness. You need to appreciate what's going on, and you need to have some practical rational understanding about it all, including the laws of mechanics. And so when you begin to think of these things in simple ways, to see what the problem is, you can then begin to understand where some obvious solutions lie. If you've got somebody who has problems with breathing, difficulties breathing, then surely you must look to see how much muscle tension they're making, particularly to hold themselves up, because that must be the major factor in the interference.

It has to be. It may not be by any means the only factor, but if you can eliminate that then at least you are free to address the other factors. And this is also a factor that you can do something about. It's something that can be addressed and can be helped.

So, from a practical point of view, you need to, first of all, find your static balance. That is to say, you're just standing still and not going anywhere. What you're doing is ensuring that you've got your full height, ensuring that you're in proper shape, ensuring that you're not doing anything through some habit or false notion that you've got. You're not holding yourself for reasons of vanity or anything else, you're leaving yourself alone, but leaving yourself alone with the intent of arriving at your proper shape and at your full height. And then in proper shape and at full height, you find the balance. Finding the balance is experimental. It's for you to judge whether you're in balance or out of balance, whether you're making more effort than is necessary, whether you can manage to reduce the amount of effort that you're making without losing height, losing shape. You'll see how little effort is necessary to stand and you will undoubtedly find that it does marvels for your breathing straight away. So, that is the start of things. That is the very beginning.

Within vertebrates, in creatures with spines, it is the head that leads and the body that follows. The head leads and the body follows. That phrase does describe what happens. But let us consider the implications of this statement. You've got the skull, and it's got a certain amount of brain inside—depending on the individual of course—and hair and tissue of one sort and another, which makes it quite heavy. And when we say it's heavy, we mean it is influenced by gravitation and therefore needs support. You've got to remember that every part of the body is influenced by gravity, and therefore every part of the body needs supporting if it isn't going to be collapsing and going down towards the earth. And the whole neuromuscular mechanism really works to support the head. The head has to be supported first off. That's the first consideration. So sagging, drooping, falling, collapsing, all that sort of thing: That's out. Absolutely. The head has got to be supported. But now, we've got to go beyond support because we've said that the head leads and the body follows.

Now if the head is going to move, if it's going to go anywhere in space, if it's actually going to go anywhere, then you've got to have freedom in the neck. If the neck is locked and fixed and rigid, then the head can't move independently. So freedom of the neck is the next requirement if the head is going to lead and the body is going to follow. But freedom of the neck by itself isn't going to do anything very much, because all the freedom of the neck is going to do by itself is let the head wobble about. It is going to be supported but it's going to be supported rather precariously, and it's going to be at risk of falling in all sorts of different directions. So if the head is going to lead somewhere, then leading means, as far as vertebrates are concerned, that there has to be an energy, a direction, a flow of energy through the spine. It is through the direction of the spine that the head leads the way. In other words, the spine is tending to lengthen. Energy is flowing along the direction of the spine. So the head leading and body following necessitates, if you think about it, that the neck has got to be free and the back's got to lengthen. The spine has got to lengthen. The torso has got to lengthen. The whole of you has got to lengthen.

So, of course, a knowledge of the bones and the muscles is important, but the most important practical consideration in studying and understanding anatomy is to understand the mechanics of the situation, to understand that the whole structure has got to find its proper shape. Then anatomy can become the study of the proper shape, the structures that underlie all the different workings, the structures that underlie the process of poise and balance, with the head leading and the body following. That's the sort of starting framework that I think is rather useful to consider.

Apart from all knowledge

I THOUGHT THIS MIGHT BE an opportunity to think a bit about the talks that we've been having over the last term and a half on anatomy, the nervous system, the stretch reflexes and the brain. Among all these different things we've built up a good picture of the working of the mechanisms of the self. To build up a really good knowledge is very valuable. At the same time, you need to pause every now and then and consider how to make the best use of it.

By next term I shall be starting to read *The Use of the Self*. We shall then be going back to a consideration of Alexander's own experiences and his attitudes and the situation in which he found himself as a young man and how the whole Technique originated and evolved. The point that we always need to remind ourselves is that he was confronted with a very real problem, and he was looking for a solution to this problem. Now, he'd already gained quite a lot of experience at the start of his career. He wasn't a complete beginner when it came to reciting and acting and so on, and the question he put to himself was: What am I doing wrong that is causing the trouble?

Now, not everybody asks that question of themselves when they are confronted with a problem or a difficulty. It doesn't occur to you to say straight away, "What am I doing wrong about it?" The first thing that usually arises is, "What ought I to do about it? Can I find somebody who can tell me what to do to put it right? How do I tackle this? What is it that I need to do?" And, if you like, "What do I need to know?" If you ask yourself what do I need to know about voice, for instance, there's no limit to what you need to know. The amount that is involved that is to be found out is absolutely enormous and you can't possibly say in advance what you really need to know.

That is the point that I want to make about the study of anatomy and physiology and psychology and all the other relevant fields of inquiry. It's no good restricting yourself and saying, "Well I don't need to know that," or, "This knowledge isn't going to be of any use to me." It may well be that some bit of information that you've got stored away that you hadn't thought was particularly relevant suddenly can be seen to apply in this particular situation and give you some new insight and some new guidance. So, I'm all for people gaining as much knowledge as they have the opportunity to gain in as many directions as possible. I wouldn't limit it at all.

On the other hand, let's go back to the question that Alexander asked himself: What am I doing wrong that is causing the trouble? Now, that's the question that is not at all easy to answer out of prior knowledge. You've really got to take an objective look at the situation. You've got to study the situation in hand, and see what you can discern about what is going on. Then from your assessment of the whole situation, you can begin to gauge what might be wrong, what might possibly be causing trouble. You can form a hypothesis, and you can test it out.

Of course the story of the evolution of the Technique is the story of thought and experience and development on those lines. If Alexander had known a great deal about the working of the postural mechanism, if he'd known about the stretch reflexes, for example, it wouldn't have given any immediate help to him in the problem that he faced because, apart from all knowledge, the fact of the matter was, as he discovered, he was doing certain things that were wrong and he was doing them as an outcome of habit. He learned that he was a creature of habit and we can all learn that we are creatures of habit. It's only when you really recognize for yourself that here is some habit that you want to change that the implications of it all begin to come home to you. But it isn't a matter then of knowledge of facts and knowledge of this and that, it's very much a knowledge of yourself, experience of your own will, your own willing and wishing. It's a very, very personal, individual thing.

Alexander soon discovered that when he went to speak he was not only making too much tension and that the tension was obviously the cause of his vocal tiredness, his loss of voice; he also realized that the tension involved what he called shortening in stature or what we familiarly refer to as pulling down. And this was an observation that he made when he went to speak—he pulled down. Now, of course, later on he came to realize that his sensory appreciation was not too reliable, that what his feelings told him was not always correct. But the observation that when he spoke he pulled down, that certainly stood up to repeated experiment. It was something that was sufficiently demonstrable not to be any doubt or argument about. It wasn't the case of him saying that he felt he pulled down or he thought he pulled down and perhaps he didn't pull down after all. No, everything confirmed that he did pull down. The trouble was that there were times when as far as his feelings were concerned he thought he'd done it all right. He hadn't noticed that there was anything wrong. It was this lack of noticing, it was this lack of awareness and observation, that then led him to the conclusion that things were all right when they weren't all right. Well, again, this is a fact that you only really become aware of through self-observation and self experiment when you start to address your own personal problems.

The question still remains: If I'm doing something wrong and if I now have a fairly good idea what it is that I am doing wrong, what am I going to do about it? And that is the very difficult question for everybody. It is a difficulty that is very much compounded by the fact that in our culture, in our education, all the emphasis in learning and teaching is learning what is the right thing to do and then finding out how to do it. The emphasis is all in that direction.

What we're discussing is what prevention actually means in this technique. Essentially, it means, on the one hand, the process whereby we give ourselves time, we prevent the automatic inevitable response, what Alexander used to refer to as the "too quick and unthinking reaction." That really says it all, a "too quick and unthinking reaction." That's what we're trying to prevent. If we can prevent the too quick and unthinking reaction, then we've got the possibility of also preventing the interference with that vital mechanism that counteracts the depressive forces of gravitation and indeed all the other depressive forces and influences that get us down. When we prevent the unfavorable reaction, we prevent the consequences of that reaction.

Now it's perfectly true you can't escape from the fact that having prevented all that there are still going to be lots and lots of problems to confront and face. When you've given yourself time to choose you can still choose the wrong thing. It's quite easy to make the wrong choices. Even when you've succeeded in stopping pulling down so that you are poised and balanced and very much in better shape altogether, you've still got things to do, you've still got things to apply yourselves to. And the old sneer of years and years ago was, when the little book on the Alexander Technique called *Knowing How to Stop* was published, people said, "Well, when's the next volume entitled *Knowing How to Proceed* coming out?"

It is perfectly true that prevention doesn't answer all the questions. It doesn't solve all the problems. The thing to realize is that it is the starting point. It is the beginning. We have to find out how to prevent the wrong thing above all, apart from whatever knowledge we can gain, whatever vision we can formulate, whatever plans we can make in all directions. That starting point is indispensable. From there we can start building our knowledge of all these different fields. And that's the relationship between what we're doing in our daily work and the lectures and learning of anatomy and physiology and all the rest of it.

A *visual impression*

THE MIRRORS ARE quite important learning tools, and they are something that we can rather neglect and take for granted.

We have the mirrors here, on the training course, but people don't use them a great deal. The difficulty is that most of us are not professional actors or professional performers. On the whole, we don't really like looking at ourselves in the mirror. Or if we do like looking in the mirror, we tend on the whole not to like what we see very much.

F.M. always believed that as students we should use mirrors, and so at Ashley Place in the little back teaching room there was a set up of mirrors, rather like in a tailor's so that you could see all four views. And we used to use the mirrors and we did find that it took quite a bit of getting used to. First, you had to get over the fright of seeing yourself. Then, you'd start noticing that you're poking your head forward, or that you've twisted yourself, or you're not standing in balance. All these things you'd notice and you'd try to fix the problem as rapidly as possible. And so just as if your hair is untidy, you'll find you'll automatically be putting a hand up, straightening it, or straightening your tie, or whatever it is, if you find that you're in some attitude, your head on one side or poking your neck forward or whatever it is, you do something about it to correct it.

Well, when you back off and think about it, you'll realize of course that that isn't the way. You can't try to fix the problem directly in that way. The proper way definitely is to say no and not do anything but pause and really continue to look at the situation, assessing the situation, and say, yes that's the way it is. And then consider what means whereby, what you're going to do to correct it. So if you are doing something like poking your neck forward and generally pulling yourself down, then you have to stop and inhibit. Then you can begin to direct and remember to release your neck.

After you've stopped yourself from making a quick fix, so to speak, the next thing is that you think, "Well now I ought to do some mirror work." So you go and sit down in front of the mirror, and you think "Now, what I'm going to do is I'm going to sit in front of the mirrors and give my orders." So you sit in front of the mirror and you say, "Neck be free, head forward and up, back lengthened and widened, knees forward and away, neck and head forward and up, back lengthened and widened, knees forward and away," and you look at yourself and naturally, at least subconsciously, you're looking for something to happen. You want to see yourself lengthening. You want to see yourself going up. You want to see a response to the orders that you've given. Since you don't see any immediate response, you can pretty well guarantee, you can bet on it, the next thing that will happen is that you will be trying to make it happen. And you will not be content with just simply thinking of the head going forward and up, you will be trying to push your head forward and up.

I do remember people who used to go and do mirror work like that, and it was an absolute disaster, because after they'd done a quarter of an hour or so of conscientious mirror work, they'd be just so stiff, you couldn't believe it. But mirror work isn't a matter of just standing there or sitting there, it's a matter of carrying out some procedure, something that involves movement, and observing as you carry it out, observing as far as you can, what happens. Not only is that more interesting and more likely to actually show you something visually, but it will also help keep you from trying to see a change happen. That can be terribly counterproductive.

I like to have a mirror where I'm teaching, and where I've got it in my teaching room is to my side so that as I'm working I can look up from time to time and I can see myself and see my pupil in the mirror. A fairly quick glance is very useful because I can easily pick up by the quick look whether I'm pulling myself down as I'm working, or, also, things that the pupil's doing, that sometimes being so close to the pupil you don't notice as easily. Whereas with the image in the mirror further away you've got a more comprehensive picture of it. So I recommend any teacher to have a mirror placed so that you can keep an eye on yourself. The mirror is a wonderful tool in this way, but you don't need to sit for periods of time staring at yourself or anything like that. It's just having it there so that you can check.

Now, two more things about the mirror before I stop. When I finished my training, I had become used to using the mirrors. I'd really found the mirrors very useful and particularly, of course, what I'd been very interested in was I found that if you had two mirrors set up so that you had a sideways view, you could not only see when you were pulling your head back and pulling yourself down, but you could get a pretty good impression of how the head was really pivoting on the end of the spine. You could really see that pivot, and you could see how the pull around the collar bone and the shoulders affected the base of the neck, the neck coming forward, that sort of thing. You could really then understand quite a lot about the mechanism and you could see what undoubtedly Alexander himself saw and described as the head going forward and up. Because when he used the words forward and up, he was describing what he saw taking place in the mirror. Now generations of pupils have come along and they've never actually seen that. They've felt it but they haven't seen it. And so, although they've come to an understanding of what the words forward and up mean, it's been very much more a sensory impression than a visual impression. But for Alexander himself, particularly initially, it was very, very much a visual impression. Before the Technique became a sensory technique, it relied very much on the visual impression.

As the Technique evolved, it became more sensory, more to do with the lengthening and the effect on the voice and the breathing and all the rest of it, so that the visual thing was rather left behind. Alexander had moved from using the mirrors and the visual cues to being able to rectify his sensory thinking. He was able to exercise better sensory judgment. But he started with the mirrors. And I think it is very useful to use the mirrors to experiment and try to see, not what you're doing right, but to try and see what you're doing wrong.

When I first started teaching, I used to like to take people and give them a lesson in front of the mirror so that I could show them, and so that they could watch themselves and see what I meant by the head being pulled back, the neck going forward. That seemed very sensible and reasonable, and it did indeed work with some people, but there were an awful lot of people upon whom it had just the opposite effect. I found that it made them so tense, it made them so nervous, that it was making it impossible to get what I wanted. Even with the ones who got some benefit from the visual impression, the visual impression wasn't particularly useful when they weren't in front of the mirror. Because when they walked away, the sensory monitoring of the situation, directing and thinking, became the primary process they had to make use of in ordinary everyday life.

And so what I'm really saying, to sum up, is yes, do try the mirrors. It is really quite interesting to think about where the Technique started. I recommend using the mirrors to anybody as something to try out, but be aware of just sitting in front of the mirror waiting to see your head go forward and up. It is a trap that is very easy to fall into.

Theory and practice

AS I'VE MENTIONED BEFORE, when Alexander started out none of the scientific work on the physiology of the postural mechanism had been attempted at all. If you look at it perfectly simply, what Alexander had seen was that people must not pull themselves down. When you go to do anything if you pull down, then that has a harmful and damaging affect on the works. What you need to do is find a way to avoid pulling down and to free and activate the mechanism that is programmed to take you up.

Now, in 1978 T.D.M. Roberts published his book called *The Neurophysiology of Postural Mechanisms*. He made the simple statement that the postural mechanisms work, and that the essence of their working is to prevent punishing collisions between our heads and the planet. So Roberts was saying that you must not pull down, and if you do pull down, harm will come. It took a long time for that to be recognized and accepted. It's an accepted theory, but people are still light years away from appreciating any of the practical implications of it.

And the same thing holds true for the first scientific

breakthrough on the Technique, which was the publication of Rudolph Magnus' findings about the significance of the head/neck relationship. Magnus had done a lot of work about the balance of the head, the attitude of the head in space, and the postural mechanisms. His findings have been summarized in the short phrase that the head leads and the body follows. The head leads and the body follows is the secret of locomotion and the secret of poise and balance and all the rest of it. Obviously, you've got lots more to say about it than that, but that was really the essence of the whole thing, and so you can imagine how excited, how thrilled Alexander was, when this all first came to light, because nobody before Magnus had ever, from a scientific point of view, shown the primary importance of the head/neck/back relationship.

So here, for the first time, was scientific confirmation of what Alexander discovered and had been working on. Alexander rather naively assumed that scientists and people working in the field and particularly people like orthopedic surgeons, medical men who were concerned with health and well-being and so on, would immediately latch onto these experiments, would see the implications of them, and revise their practical ideas and practical procedures in accordance with the new scientific discoveries. Of course, we all know very well things don't happen like that. In most fields, in practically all fields, it takes years and years and years before a new scientific discovery filters down to a level where anybody is even entertaining the idea of doing anything about it from a practical point of view.

Why is any of this information practical today? Why rehearse all this old history? The practical answer that appeals to me is that in our work as teachers of this technique, we are very much concerned with what people think. We're concerned with what people think and how they think. What information, and in what form, will really change people's thinking, their thought processes? It's only by that sort of study that you've got the possibility of seeing how you can influence it, how you can swing it to get people to think a little but more usefully, a little bit more practically and productively. It is all about the way you and I think, and the way other people think. That's what it's really all about. And when you see what Magnus laid out, what T.D.M. Roberts laid out, and realize how little people's practical views have changed, you can see that you have your work cut out for you to get people to think in a new way.

Spinal curvature

PEOPLE ALWAYS THINK of spinal curvature as a medical or pathological condition. And so it very often is. But what we need to bear in mind is that when we pull ourselves down, we tend to develop spinal curvature. If you don't want that spinal curvature, the thing is not to pull yourself down. There are, of course, pathological and genetic causes of spinal curvature, but those are at the extremes. The tendency towards spinal curvature is pretty well universal. And it's universally something that we want to avoid if we possibly can.

By spinal curvature I mean the distortion of the spine usually thought of in terms of lateral curvature or scoliosis. If you look at pictures of the spine, a straight spine viewed either from the front or the back appears in a straight line, not curved. If you look at it sideways then you see that it has what we call natural curves—the small curve of the neck, the larger of the back, the bigger curve of the lower back, a curve of the sacrum and the coccyx curve as well. So, looking at it from the side you've got those curves and those are, so to speak, normal curves. And then, if someone wants to represent what is called scoliosis, it is represented in a picture either from the front or the back and you see that instead of having a vertical line you've got a line with a squiggle in it. It distorts sideways.

But these are all pictures. These are all figments of the imagination. If you look at a skeleton or if you look at another person, you'll see that it's a three dimensional thing. And in three dimensions, quite simply, when the whole structure starts to curve, it tends to corkscrew. It's not just a simple matter of fore, aft and lateral curves; it's a three dimensional thing. When you pull down, what is tending to happen is that the spine is shortening. It is losing overall length, and in doing so it is tending to corkscrew. Now, since we are not dealing with it from a medical point of view or a physiotherapy point of view or osteopathy or anything like that, we're not concerned to look to see how you're corkscrewing. Our primary concern is to avoid doing so. And the avoidance of shortening, of corkscrewing, can involve all kinds of considerations, but the main thing is the simple realization that if you interfere with the natural mechanism that takes you up, then when that mechanism is interfered with you tend to come down and shorten. When you shorten, you go into a corkscrew.

Few people have really given any thought and consideration to how you use the spine and the back. Let me give a simple, everyday example: You are going to pick something up on the ground, or you're going to reach up above your head. Obviously, when you do those things it affects the spine. Now what you need to observe is: What effect does it have? Does it cause distortion in such a way that you get a build-up of pressure on some of the spinal joints? Is all the pressure focused in one or two areas? Or is it possible to do what you want in such a way that the work is distributed over the whole spine so that all the joints in the spine, all the bits, do their share of work? Of course, the spine is still taking load, it's doing work, it's resisting tension and pressure, but it's doing it in such a way that it's maintaining its own wholeness, its own integrity. It's not suffering from extreme stress in one bit whereas another bit is doing nothing. You can be absolutely certain that from the point of view of design and construction the spine is supposed to share out the work so that every bit of the spine contributes its share. If it doesn't, if each bit doesn't do its appropriate share, then some bits get overloaded and other bits get underloaded and you get damage.

Now, if the spine gets twisted and distorted, that will affect the rib cage and the internal capacity of the thoracic area will be very much decreased. And one of the main practical considerations in life is that you don't want to reduce this internal capacity any more than is absolutely unavoidable. On the contrary, your best interests lie in increasing the internal capacity here as much as you can for the simple reason that if you've got more room here you've got more power to breathe. But it isn't just the breathing. Compression, pulling down, twisting, seriously interfere with the whole works; it's only through having as much internal capacity as possible, as much freedom as possible, reducing the pressure as far as you can, that you lighten the burden on the heart, on the lungs, on the circulatory system and on the entire system.

Looking at all of this from a practical teaching situation, I have a pupil who has got a curvature, so I'm taking the head and neck and I'm freeing the neck as I take the head forward and up. I'm encouraging the lengthening and getting the pupil to think of the lengthening, but at the same time, with my hands on the thorax, I'm feeling the twist and I'm seeing if I can just give a bit of encouragement to untwist the spine by widening a bit. And when that happens, we get a bit more lengthening. So, what one is always doing is working to get the lengthening and the widening. And you've got to watch it because if you get too enthusiastic about the lengthening so that the pupil joins in and starts trying to help you, which is very likely to happen, then you detect that at once because the torso will start fixing and narrowing.

Of course, it can happen that things seem to be going okay and you're working on the torso, and you feel you are getting a bit of expansion, and the ribs are beginning to move. But you look up at the head and you realize that the head is sinking into the neck like a blessed tortoise. So that's no good either. What you've got to do from a practical working point of view is when you work at the torso, make sure that you're not losing length or getting stiffness at the head and neck. And if you're working on the head and neck, then watch to see that you're not getting fixing and narrowing in the ribs, the back, the entire torso. So you're always using one against the other so to speak. You're working on one and watching the other. The other is your check. And F.M. used to say that this was one of the great practical beauties of the Technique. You can't make a mistake if you watch to see that the widening is taking place as you're getting the lengthening, and if you make sure that the lengthening is taking place as you get the widening. If you really observe those two processes, you can't make a mistake.

The biggest practical problem we face in our teaching is not a particular twist or pull, it is indeed the erroneously preconceived ideas the pupil holds that are the main stumbling blocks. And the most common erroneously preconceived idea, the most predominant of all, is the idea that you've got to do something. If the pupil, the person that you're working on, believes in doing, believes that they've got to do something then they will try to help you. If you indicate that you want length, they'll try to lengthen. If you indicate that you want widening, they'll try to widen. You can be quite sure that when you look at them, and look at them with their curvature and their shortening, that except for the extreme cases we mentioned at the outset, these twists and curves are associated with their ideas and beliefs.

Ironically, the underlying misunderstanding, the underlying problem, is that they haven't realized and appreciated that they are the possessors of a very sophisticated and complex mechanism which is expressly designed to do whatever they want to do. Practically, whatever they want to be done the mechanism is expressly designed to do it. But the mechanism has got to have the correct instructions. People don't worry about that, what they do is they try to force the mechanism to work regardless of how the mechanism is designed to work, and how it is in fact working. And that is the one thing that keeps them from getting the mechanism to do what they want. They create the interference and then think that the problem is with the mechanism itself. Not true, not true at all.

The primary wish

WE USE THE TERM primary control in our work. *The Universal Constant in Living* is really the book in which the phrase "primary control" comes to be used such a lot. You won't find the term primary control in *Man's Supreme Inheritance* or in the second book, *Constructive Conscious Control*. The reason is not that Alexander wasn't aware of the primary control or he hadn't discovered it or something of that kind. In his experience and working and teaching, he hadn't up to that time found the words that he thought would be most useful to use to describe the underlying experience and the concept. And from his standpoint, and I suppose you could say from ours, the phrase primary control is very handy. It's a very good simple label that you can put on and make use of. But to people who haven't had the experience and therefore haven't got a similar understanding, the phrase is not only useless but can also be quite misleading.

Now from our experience we can say that the head and the neck, the working of all the neuromuscular apparatus, regulates the whole matter of balance and coordinates the working of the musculature so that quite simply we are able to move around without falling over. It is undoubtedly the head/neck/back relationship that is the central agency, the primary agency if you like, whereby the whole apparatus works so that you don't fall over, you don't collapse, you don't sink down.

Obviously this is something that is extremely complex, but there are two things we can say about it quite safely. One is that the resultant of all the activity is movement in an upward direction. If the body didn't generate movement in an upward direction, it wouldn't be able to counteract gravitation. The head is always moving upwards. The total effect is that upward movement is being generated not only as far as the head is concerned but as far as the whole body is concerned.

In science, in physiology, they talk about supporting reactions. The physiologists are very much inclined to describe these supporting mechanisms in rather a fixed way so that it's just certain muscle contractions—for instance, a lock of the knee joints or a lock of the ankle joints or shoulder joints—that keep the joints from suddenly folding and collapsing underneath you. Such responses are called supporting reactions. But when you look into the neurology of it, and you look beyond the mere muscle action, you can see that you've got something much more mobile going on. The supporting reaction is a very positive process of generating movement, generating a flow of energy that is counterbalancing the other downward forces. So you've got an upward direction.

You can say the primary direction is up. It's primary because it's absolutely the first consideration. If there isn't the up, you're in trouble. In *Man's Supreme Inheritance*, if you comb through it very carefully, you will find that Alexander uses the phrase "the primary movement." Alexander wasn't concerned with the anatomy or physiology of the primary movement, but he was very much concerned with the practical reality that if a primary movement wasn't taking place, then his breathing was interfered with, his voice was interfered with, and all sorts of things were going wrong.

Now in order that an upward movement shall take place, there has to be an interaction of the body's musculature. In other words, all the different muscles have got to be working together to produce this end product. How they all work, how the interplay works, is vastly complicated. But you can see that if you've got some muscles that are too tense, if some are too slack, if you haven't got the whole thing regulated and coordinated, then you're not going to achieve the primary movement. So the primary movement depends on the regulation of the muscle tone. If you haven't got that regulation then you don't have the movement. We can say quite definitely that we've got a regulator there and it is primary—primary in the sense that that's what's got to happen first of all in order to get the movement. But then it comes back to you.

It is your muscles. It is you that has got to move upwards. So it's your choice. It's got to be your wish.

Clearly, if you don't wish it, especially if you really wish something contradictory, if you really want to stiffen, if you've got a good dose of the death wish, then there's really nothing to stop your wishes being fulfilled and carried out. So we come back again to something primary. We come back to a primary wish. It's a primary wish in order that energy may be generated to produce a primary movement up. You exercise the control over the whole apparatus through your willing and wishing. You are exercising a control primarily, or a primary control, over a primary set of conditions that are going to produce a primary result.

So I'm only just referring to the very simple outline of it. You could elaborate it a great deal farther and if you go into it in detail, more elaboration will occur to you. But to deal with complex and elaborate things we do need a simple label, and that is what the label primary control is for. But if you don't see the practical implications of this term, then primary control is non-meaning or, at worse, it can be seen to mean some curious little box of tricks, some sort of black box that has an entirely mythological existence. It can be taken over and adopted as some device that you can use by doing something with it, as if it is something separate from yourself. Unfortunately, this is what many people have been looking for all along.

So there you have it. Yes, let's use the term primary control. But let's bear in mind that the primary part of this control is your wish and intent. The rest flows from that.

Forward and up

THIS WHOLE BUSINESS about the relation-
ship between the head and the neck is crucial. There is so
much to understand and to think about, and there's so
much that is misunderstood, even among fairly experienced Alexander teachers. In my training, Alexander
talked about the head moving forward and up, and he
took your head in his hands and showed you what was
meant by this. As lessons progressed, you got more and
more an experience and an impression of the process.
You got to know what it felt like, and therefore better
understood what it was all about.

But the anatomy and the physiology of the situation
was something else. We didn't really know much about
that. Alexander said in *The Use of the Self* that the head
has got to go forward and up. And so we all believed that
that was what it was all about. You've got to direct your
own head forward and up, and if you were a teacher, it
was your job to take other people's heads forward and
up. But what was this forward and up? What is this forward and up, what does it really mean?

As I've said to you before, lots of people reading *The*

Use of the Self for the first time would go and look in the mirror and they would try it out and say, "Well, that's my head going forward, and up must be up there somewhere." And they would pull and lift and get themselves into quite a state. Further thought and observation led people to go back and look at the book again. They would rediscover that Alexander said that what you mustn't do is pull the head back; the head mustn't be pulled back. He also said, if you go and look at the book very carefully, that you mustn't shorten in stature, you mustn't, as we say, come down. When you pull the head back, it's fairly evident that shortening takes place. The more you pull the head back, the more you're inclined to shorten.

So the opposite of shortening is lengthening. The opposite of back and down is forward and up. Unfortunately, this doesn't go very far in shedding light on what is actually involved, what the head going forward and up is all about. Now, as anatomical knowledge is gradually spread around and people have seen more, they've realized that shortening in stature is not a good idea because if you shorten in stature you distort the whole framework of the body. Even quite an elementary understanding of mechanics makes you realize that standing in an upright position, standing in an upright attitude, involves being as nearly vertical as you possibly can. You need to be balanced or poised in the vertical, and any leaning, twisting, sagging, departing from the vertical inevitably means that much more energy is going to be needed to hold yourself up. So if you're going to have a chance of being free and mobile as you stand up, you really do need to lengthen rather than shorten. The more you encourage lengthening, the more you will tend towards verticality and balance and uprightness.

When we look at the head on the end of the spine, and take in the anatomical details of the situation, it is clear that the head has got to go in an upwards direction. It has got to go up in such a manner that the relativity with the spine is not changed. That is to say, you don't want the head either to tilt backwards or tilt forwards as it goes up. If you're lengthening, and really getting to your full height, the head has got to continue upwards without tilting backwards or tilting forwards. It goes in a vertical direction. When, however, you come to put all this into practice and see how it's going to happen, you find that one of the practical difficulties is that the head is sitting on that top joint in such a way that the head would fall forward without the neck muscles in back. It would fall down towards the chest because that's where the weight of the head is—more of the weight of the head is in front. So when the head is poised on the end of the spine, you have a situation in which there are antagonistic forces in operation. There is the force of gravitation operating in front, and there's the force exerted by the neck muscles that counteract that downward fall. So you've got an equation there between two forces.

Now we said we want to go up, so quite clearly we must counteract the downward force sufficiently to avoid going down in front. But on the other hand, if you overdo the counteraction of the downward force by generating more energy in the neck, that clearly will have the effect of tilting the head back, which is not what you want for many, many reasons—the two main ones being that you're no longer in balance and you're shortening in stature.

So, it's not too difficult to understand what is meant by pulling the head back. Generally speaking it means that the head is being tilted backwards on the atlantal occipital joint, on the top joint. The head is being tilted back and that is what is meant by pulling the head back, and we don't want to do it. But the up, the forward and up if you like, the lengthening in stature, that I'm afraid inevitably has to remain a bit of a mystery.

Nobody really knows at the present time exactly how the whole neuromuscular mechanism, how the neurophysiology, works. How it is that throughout the whole organism the energy is generated to neutralize the gravitational effect? You see, even with the tremendous amount of study that has been made in quite recent years into the neurophysiology of the postural mechanisms, it's something that is still too complex to admit a simple explanation and really simple understanding. We don't really know how it works. We do know, however, that it works.

And don't forget it works in everybody so long as

they're alive. It's just a question of how efficiently it's working. If it didn't work at all, you would be an inert heap on the floor. And insofar as you're not an inert heap on the floor, you can say that the mechanism is working to some extent. You have to accept the fact that this mechanism does work. People do go up. People go up more at some times and in some circumstances than others. There's a very big variation and clearly it is desirable that you should go up as much as possible all the time. Because the more the upward energy flows, the lighter and freer you'll be, and the more that all the functioning of the body—respiration, circulation, digestion—is able to operate. Putting it the other way round, the less you go up, the more you pull down, the heavier you become and the more the respiration, circulation, digestion are handicapped and suffer for it.

So that's all pretty straightforward. We've established then that the need is to go up, that the machinery is there seeking to do it, and of course, it was Alexander's practical understanding that, as he put it quite simply, "the right thing does itself." In other words, the machinery will work, if it's not interfered with. You don't have to do anything about it other than to free it, to want it to work, and to let it work.

But when we come to looking at the anatomical and physiological detail of things, although we don't know how it works, we are able to discern things that interfere with the working. We can identify certain processes, cer-

tain activities, as very definitely wrong. Alexander pointed out that you mustn't tilt the head back. But when
you look at the majority of people standing, for instance,
you will see that the most obvious thing about their
length is that the neck is inclined forward, that the neck
is out of alignment with the rest of the spine. The neck
is being drawn forward at an angle. You're not lengthening, you're not gaining your full height, if your neck is
poking forward.

When the neck pokes forward, there's a very practical
reason why the head will tilt backwards on the neck, and
that is that you want to hold your head up and be able to
look around. If your neck pokes forward and you keep
the same relativity between the head and neck, you'll
find that your head is down and you're looking at the
floor all the time which, naturally, you don't want to do.
So you've got good practical reasons for pulling your
head back.

What is really happening is people are trying to hold
the head up but at the same time they are, unawares,
exerting quite a lot of muscular effort that is pulling the
neck forward and down. In other words, they're trying to
do two things at the same time. They're doing something
wrong, and then trying to correct it by doing something
else. There's a battle there. And what we say in the Technique, from a practical point of view, is first of all, stop
pulling your neck forward, and then if you stop pulling
your neck forward, it must be fairly easy to coax it back

into proper place, into proper alignment. And when you get your neck back into proper alignment, you won't have the need to pull your head back, you won't want to pull your head back.

Frank Pierce Jones, in one of his papers, drew attention to the very significant anatomical detail that from the so-called mastoid process, those bumps on the skull behind the ears, you have the sternocleidomastoid muscles coming down the sides of the neck to the collar bones and the top of the breast-bone. When these muscles, acting together, tighten and shorten they draw everything forward and down. Since they are attached to the skull behind the joint on which the head pivots they will, at the same time, pull the head back. Thus when the neck is drawn forward under the influence of these sternocleidomastoid muscles, the head is inevitably pulled back.

Now what Frank Pierce Jones was saying about that is important to bear in mind. It's the pull down in front that is mainly responsible for pulling your head back. Yes, the muscles in the back, when they tighten, can tilt the head back also. There are lots of ways in which you can pull your head back, but the commonest way of pulling down and pulling your head back is the shortening and contraction that follows through the sternocleidomastoid specifically, and, more generally, through all the different parts that are in front.

So you can see that the neck must be free to bring about the balance of the head. If the neck is pulled forward, the head will be pulled back. Freedom of the neck is the keynote because it's only when you've got that freedom can the energy flow occur that is necessary for uprightness or counteraction of gravity. Without that freedom, the postural balance is no longer finely tuned.

So you do have a very, very practical reason for thinking and directing, ordering, wishing your neck to be free. If your neck isn't free, the possibility of your head going forward and up doesn't exist. The neck has got to be free. It is the foundation. Unfortunately, in the case of practically all of us, it is not habitually free. When it is not free, the head is tilted slightly backwards. The consequence of releasing the neck will be to correct the balance of the head on the neck. Rather than having to move the head into a "forward" position, the backward tilt will not take place when the neck is free, and the head will automatically move slightly forward in response. Then the head can achieve an attitude of equilibrium. And then, and only then, can uprightness work.

Knees forward and away

I THOUGHT THIS MORNING I would talk a bit about legs and feet, and focus on the old familiar directions of "knees forward and away." People parrot the phrase "knees forward and away" and I don't think many people understand what the words mean or why they are used.

The two things to understand are, first of all, that "knees forward and away" is a preventive order. It is not to make certain things happen. It is to prevent certain other things happening. Alexander emphasizes in *The Use of the Self* the importance of preventive orders, but people don't really understand what that means. You see, the problem should be pretty familiar because I think in the back of everybody's mind you get people saying, "Here's the right thing, I want the knees to go forward and away, so it is up to me to make it happen. What is preventive in that?" This is where I want to start looking at the situation.

Take a look at a child of three or four and you see that when they go to squat there is a definite spiral or rotation action in the legs which you can describe as the knees going forward and away. If you don't know what I mean, take the first opportunity you get to look at a child of that age and you'll see. The knees do go forward. They go forward over the feet and ankles, but they also go apart and the action of the muscles is a spiral action. It is what we call external rotation.

As I've said, that is the norm. You might say that is what we want to happen. But having agreed that is what we want to happen, let us look at something that is very much more important and significant—what we don't want to happen. Now when you look at it physiologically you find that the adductor muscles of the thighs, the inside muscles that pull the knees together, are very strong and very active. It is like the knees are being drawn towards the pelvis but it is in fact more like the pubic symphysis being drawn towards the knees. There is a tremendous shortening right through the inside—the pelvic floor and the butt muscles are all contracted. You can generate a marvelous amount of tension if you really make a good job of it. You can make massive tension there which has the effect of internally rotating the thighs, pulling the legs together, drawing the knees back and locking the whole thing up. That is what we don't want.

So, at the outset, never mind what we do want. Everybody thinks that what we do want is what matters, but of course it isn't. The thing that matters is what we don't want. If we can be clear about what we don't want, what mustn't take place, then we can watch out and at the very first signs that it is going wrong, we can quickly intervene and, hopefully, stop it. But people's minds don't work in that way. They are so darn concerned with getting it right—they know what ought to happen, that the knees ought to work like the little child, it ought to be like that—they never notice, they never pay attention to what is really happening. They never pick up the early signs of things going wrong at all. By the time they do notice that things are going wrong, they've gone wrong and it is too late.

By getting people to focus on the knees going forward and away, you should prevent, to a certain extent, them internally rotating, tightening, and drawing the legs together. The only trouble is that when you suggest this preventive order of the knees going forward and away, they will try and do it. The consideration for you as a teacher is how can we manage to help the pupil, to change the pupil's attitude. Of course the pupil, as we were saying yesterday, will do what they feel to be right. They use their legs in a way in which they feel happy and secure and confident.

The way that people actually use their legs, what they actually do, is habitual, the product of any number of different factors and influences of which they are liable to be totally unaware when they come to you for lessons. You can see that they are using the legs all wrong and you've got to start to make change in the way that they use their legs. As you do begin to make change, you will find that you run up against all sorts of resistances that arise from their feelings. There is also quite a mental resistance to change. Sometimes, they even gain a sort of "eureka" experience when they suddenly find that the ankle and foot can be free and that they can use it in a totally different way. That is splendid except for the fact that they get so involved with that change, they start thinking more about their foot than about their head and their general use of themselves. They start doing a specific thing with the foot and, in the process, overlook the total pattern.

As a teacher, you've got all these different factors and considerations. What I've been trying out just lately with various people is this idea: I talk to them about their feet and the contact of the foot on the ground and what I put to them quite simply is the same thing that Sally Swift, the riding instructor, was talking about when she was in here the other day. You remember she was saying that under the sole of the foot, behind the toes, there is a point that as far as acupuncture is concerned is connected to the balance of the body. As an aside, people who do tightrope walking find it absolutely necessary to have the foot in contact with the rope so that the heel is on the rope and this point just behind the toes is in contact with the rope. It is only when the heel and that part of the foot are in contact that you will get the sensory feedback necessary for keeping your balance.

What Sally Swift said was that according to Newton a force in one direction generates an equal and opposite force in the opposite direction. So you've got the weight of your body going down onto the floor. The floor then generates a counteractive force against your foot. Using this idea, if you, as you stand, think about releasing the front part of your foot, and you think about the force from the floor that is sort of pushing up under the front part of your foot, then two practical things follow from it. One very important one is that if you really want this to happen then clearly you mustn't go stiffening your feet and tensing them and so on. If you go and make a bunch of tension in your feet you're not going to feel anything at all so you'd better free and soften your feet and free and soften this front part. If you are going to free and soften the front part then it means that obviously the heels are going to come more into contact with the ground because after all the weight has got to go somewhere.

If you stand there and let the front part of your feet be freer, then you will find that automatically that will make you fall back onto your heels. Being more back on your heels, all the muscles of the foot and the toes can be freer. The joints can be freer. You can get a better freedom of the foot and more sensitive contact with the floor. You will find that as your weight shifts more onto the heels it is really necessary to free your neck and let your head go forward and up some more. If you don't make the adjustment right throughout your head and your neck, the shift on your feet will cause you to stiffen and pull the back in and do all sorts of funny things. You've really got to watch your primary control to free the neck and get the proper relativity working in order to adjust to the consequences of your thoughts and intent to have the weight a little bit more on the heels and the feet freer.

At the same time as that, do bear in mind that where we all start is the requirement for, as Alexander put it, "lengthening in stature;" in other words, energizing towards your full height. Now when people think of energizing towards their full height, they think of the head and the neck and they can see the idea that you don't want to be shortening and curving your neck. You want the neck to lengthen. You want your back to lengthen. You want your spine to lengthen and so on. Now what about the legs? People very often have an idea, particularly with knees forward and away, that they mustn't stiffen their legs, that they mustn't brace the knees back. Of course they are right, but at the same time that means that then they think to themselves, "Well, just in order to avoid stiffening the legs and bracing the knees back, I'll just let the knees go a bit slack, I'll just let them go a little bit bendy." If you do that, you're not getting your full height.

There must be a relativity throughout all the joints where one thing is stacked up on top of the other. That is your full height. Any departure from that is not your full height. You depart from the full height by bending your knees. You depart from the full height by bracing your knees back. If the knees have locked back you are not at your full height; if your knees bend you are not at your full height. So, yes, you have got problems in determining where your legs are when they are at their full height. As far as you are concerned consciously the problem is insoluble. You haven't got a sensory means of saying, "Now I am using my legs in a way so that they are producing the full height." That is something that your whole nervous system has got to sort out.

You have to have the overall intent of going up. And you have got to make sure that you are not bracing the knees, not tightening the adductor muscles, not tightening the muscles at the pelvis and so on. You've got to take care not to do those things. Now it will probably help you to think of the knees going forward and away, but do watch out because if you've got a yen to do it, to force the knees forward and away, then you will be in trouble. So, remember, the knees forward and away is a preventive, preventive, preventive order.

Walking

VERY OFTEN WHEN anatomists and physiologists and people talk about walking, they talk about the propelling force of gravitation. What they say is that it's simply a matter, as you stand there, of allowing yourself to fall forward. Then the reflex mechanism can be brought into operation so that instinctively, or automatically, you put a foot out to save yourself from falling; and then as the foot in front goes down and you continue to allow the force of gravity to operate, you fall forward again and you put out another foot to save you. And so you are falling forward all the time and preventing yourself from a serious fall by putting a foot out in front.

That description of walking is unfortunately all too common and all too true. You can hear and see how very heavily many people step. They really do bang their feet on the ground because they really are falling forward all the time and doing what I've just described. Whereas, of course, what is desirable is to be able to step as lightly as possible and that means to maintain as much upward direction as you can. So what you've got to think of first of all is that we've only got two feet and therefore you are going to stand on one to move the other. People think of standing on the front foot to move the back foot. But it is just the opposite. As you are preparing to walk, the weight is thrown largely upon the rear foot. That is to say the body is back, your neck is free and the head is going forward and up. So from the point of view of the head, the head is leading the way, but the weight is largely on the rear foot.

Now since you're standing on the rear foot, standing largely on the back leg, that of course is taking the pressure off the front leg which is free enough to permit the knee to bend so that the foot can be lifted and placed lightly forward onto the ground. At the same time, the ankle of the rear foot bends, allowing the body to incline slightly forward, thus transferring the weight onto the front foot which now becomes the supporting leg. The rear knee is now free to bend and thus the foot is lifted but placed in front where in due course it again serves as the supporting leg so that the other foot can move forwards. As you stand thus, lengthening and widening and going up, there is this propelling force of gravitation working, but it is working not to throw you forward in such a way that you are in danger of falling, but simply so that you move from one foot to the other in a way that is quite light and free and mobile. The whole of the body is directed upwards rather than downwards and when we talk about the whole body being inclined forward from the ankle, as that process takes place, the process of inclining forward is a process of going forward and up, rather than forward and down. A small but critical difference.

Remember quite simply that in starting to walk it is the front leg that is the one that is going to move first. It is the rear leg that is to act as the support. Weight is only transferred when the front foot is in contact with the ground. That is what people get confused about and they tend to do the exact opposite of what they should do. This very much applies in the matter of walking up stairs, for instance, where it is the back foot that gives the support. We lengthen from the back foot in order to place the front foot on the step and, having placed the front foot on the step, it's from the back foot that you lengthen and raise and so the body is carried upwards; whereas what people tend to do is place the front foot on the step and then try and straighten that leg so that the work of lifting the body is all done by the front leg instead of the main work being done by the lengthening of the back leg and springing off the back leg. It is a misconception that really makes the act of walking a great deal more difficult than it has to be.

Everything flows

THE WHOLE PROCESS OF THINKING, of really getting your mind working, is not easy. It takes a lot of time. To most pupils, when they first have lessons, and for quite a long time afterwards, feelings dominate. Feelings very largely take over. Gradually, people learn to calm themselves, quiet themselves. They learn to give themselves more time so that they get the benefit from the inhibition.

Then gradually, gradually the consideration arises of what you really do want, what is really supposed to happen. You're getting a bit more objective so the orders, the directions, begin to have more positive meaning. You know you don't want to pull your head back. You do want your neck to be free, and yes, you do want your head to go forward and up and you do want to lengthen and so on. But at this stage it is still quite possible, in fact it very easily happens, that you start giving some directions, you start thinking a bit objectively, but you don't necessarily get it all into sequence. There's too much distraction, so you start thinking of freeing your neck and then you start thinking, "Well, perhaps I'm standing with the weight too much on the front part of my feet." You probably are, but if you're really going to project the directions consciously in the right sequence, then the sequence, the right sequence, inescapably is the neck first, and then the head, and then the back, and then the legs. And it has to go that way. Your head can't go as it's required if your neck is stiff. Your back can't lengthen if you're pulling your head back. Your knees can't go forward and away if you're doing things with your neck and your back and so on. So, it has to be in the sequence, and the challenge is getting to the point where you can project the directions in proper sequence, and that takes time.

It is fairly obvious that if you are looking for a coordinated integrated result, and if your attitude is an objective attitude, an observant attitude in which you know what you want, then in your projection of the orders, you will be projecting them in the relationship, in the order, that does produce a coordinated result. The whole thing has to be in sequence and order, otherwise it just won't work.

You will get a pupil who is really quite intelligent and has gone quite a way in understanding what's what, and they say, "Yes I've got to lengthen and my head has got to go forward." But they forget to remember to inhibit. What they particularly forget to remember is that the head can't go forward and up until you've freed the neck, but because they have the idea of the importance of lengthening and going up and the head leading, they're sort of rushing on from there and rushing on with that thought before they've given themselves time to ensure that they're freeing to begin with.

In life, very, very often you find yourself doing things that you didn't mean to do, that you didn't intend to do. Upon any sort of reflection and awareness, you'd be horrified at the idea that you were doing it. Well, what we are saying is that you can discover through this technique that it is possible not to do what you don't want to do. You can refuse to do what you don't want to do. You do have the possibility of stopping off what is undesirable and unwanted to you. Never mind how anybody else feels about it, we're talking about you personally. If you don't want to do it, you don't have to. And that is really the thing. That's the essence of the whole business.

There are all sorts of difficulties that people experience in coming to this realization. One of the difficulties of course is that people in their education, in their experience of life, feel that they've got to make effort. They feel they've got to try harder. If they don't, if they don't do things, by which they mean make effort and try and so on, then nothing will happen. This sort of doing, as they understand doing, of course, involves a tremendous amount of muscular effort. Trying harder means, above all, increased muscular effort. F.M. used to say to people very often, "Now, tell me, what's the difference between when you go to do something and when you try to do it?" And the difference is that when people try to do something, they make a great deal more muscular effort about it. The muscular effort is associated with an emotional attitude as well—an attitude of anxiety, fear of failure, and all that sort of thing.

So the people's experience of doing, experience of activity in that way, is often quite a stumbling block. It's really quite difficult because then you tell a pupil not to do, and in their understanding, that is either interpreted as, "All right, I won't get out of the chair, in fact I won't let you take me out of the chair. In fact, nobody's going to move me out of the chair." And so the determination not to do expresses itself in a very positive counteractive form of doing. Otherwise, of course, with their prior experience of relaxation, people respond by sort of switching off the energy and allowing themselves to slump and sag, and get into a comparatively inert state. And again, when you look at it, that is really a form of doing. It's counter productive. It's not what you want.

I think that if you really want to have a clearer picture of this concept, it was the old Greek philosopher Heracleitus who said, "Everything flows." Indeed, everything does flow. As life goes on, life flows, energy flows. You don't have to do anything to make the energy flow, you can't make the energy flow, but you can interfere with it, you can prevent it, you can stop it and also you can direct it and redirect it.

If you think of a stream of water flowing, you can

direct the water this way or that way, you can, with a bit of care and luck, stop it from flowing where you don't want it to flow—although this is often pretty difficult, as people will know if they've ever tried to do it in a practical way, because when water is flowing there's no question it, so to speak, has a life of it's own. And if you particularly don't want it to go somewhere, you've got to inhibit its flow of direction very efficiently, very effectively. With some thought and skill and care, you can get the water to flow in the direction that you want it to flow.

So this metaphor of flowing water really does give you a picture of what inhibition and direction is all about, because the problem is not the flow of energy. The problem is how you deal with it and how you control it. Of course, when people are very ill, when they're in a very exhausted condition, there are times when the energy level is very low. But even when the flow of energy is reduced because of fatigue and illness, the control of the flow is still important because if you haven't got much of it, you certainly want to get it flowing in the chosen direction and you don't want it to go to waste. Alternatively, sometimes you can have a great abundance of energy, and when there's an awful lot of energy flying about then again you've got the same problem, that is to say, the problem of making sure of the direction, because when there's masses of energy about the place, if it gets misdirected, disaster really can follow.

So strong or weak, it doesn't really signify, you're back to the same requirements of direction and control. That's really what it amounts to in the end.

Working the wheel

As ALEXANDER ALWAYS used to say, there is no such thing as breathing as such. The whole of you is involved in your breathing process. Every cell in your body has an interest in what's happening with your breathing. It is a total activity that includes your thoughts, your feelings and your emotions. And when I say it's an activity, it is, of course, a matter of movement.

Now, in order to understand how it works and how it's supposed to work, I find it useful to forget about humans and think for a moment about animals. For instance, the horse in the picture over the mantelpiece there. In the picture, you can see that the horse's spine is in the horizontal and the horse is moving forward with the head leading. That means the spine is being lengthened. It is being stretched. One of the basic instructions that is always given in riding schools and with horses is, "Ride your horse forward." Encourage the horse to go forward. The forward movement of the horse has the effect of lengthening the spine. When you consider the spine, similar to our spines with the discs and all the joints and so on, clearly if you get the horse going forward and the spine lengthening, you're taking pressure off the discs, you're taking pressure off the joints, so that the whole structure is more mobile. It's more elastic. It's more free. Whereas, if you do the opposite, you tighten and compress and shorten. Then everything, instead of getting mobile and free, gets fixed and stiff. So in the horse the critical thing is the lengthening of the spine as the horse goes forward.

When a horse is racing, when it's galloping, it is quite interesting to observe the expansion and contraction of the rib cage of the horse. This expansion and contraction is geared to the forward motion of the horse and the limbs—when the foreleg strikes the ground, the horse breathes out. When the hind leg then comes forward underneath, the horse breathes in. So it is the lengthening of the spine, the forward action, that works the breathing.

Now, so it is with us. Our spines don't lengthen in the horizontal, they lengthen in the vertical. The first requirement of a spine in the vertical plane is that there's got to be a flow of energy, a flow of muscular energy that is counterbalancing the force of gravitation. Gravitation is taking everything down and this neuromuscular activity is taking the whole of us in the opposite direction. In doing so you get the lengthening of the spine. You get the pressure taken off the discs and the joints. You get more than that because when you get the lengthening, it affects all the muscles that work the ribs.

You've got to remember that here are all these bones and they're all, as it were, clothed in muscle, and the function of muscle is first of all to gather all the bones together, to hold them in place. The fundamental point is that muscles are like springs, they're spring loaded so that they can compress and then they can come back.

The first response of the lengthening, or going up, is, as we say in our jargon, the widening. When I take your head forward and up the back lengthens. And as we take your head forward and up, and if we get the lengthening, so we get the widening because the ribs expand. The lengthening encourages the widening. The initial effect of that lengthening is to take pressure off, but it's also to stretch the muscles, the extensor muscles of the rib cage. All the extensor muscles are activated by the action of coming up, so that they contract and they lift the ribs upwards and outwards. So it's the action of going up that causes the ribs to move upwards and outwards. They move upwards and outwards and of course there is your expansion. When you get your expansion, atmospheric pressure does its stuff and air is taken in.

So what we're saying is that the upward direction, the energy that is flowing, that is lengthening the spine all the time, has the effect, first of all, of stimulating the expansion and then as this direction continues, it stimulates the contraction, and then as it continues it stimulates the expansion and contraction. The upward direction creates the conditions through which free expansion and contraction can occur.

Constant direction works the movement. In the horse it's fairly obvious, particularly in a horse that's racing. But it is basically the same with us, and this is what is not generally realized, it's not generally appreciated. Alexander realized from his observation and his experiment on himself that in order to free his breathing, to get it working with full efficiency, the primary consideration was to go up—not to stiffen the neck, not to pull the head back of course, we know all about that, but the effect was, you had to go up, you had to keep your length. Keeping the length is not a static thing, it's a dynamic process. It is ensuring that the energy flows all the time. In other words, you've got to want to do it. If you don't want to do it, there's no particular reason why it should happen. If the horse doesn't want to go forward, it can stay still.

It's perfectly possible for us to not only pull down, but to stop going anywhere in particular because we can fix ourselves. But fixation is not a good idea where breathing is concerned. That's how you hold the breath, you fix—that's what you do. So breathing is all about movement. How do you promote movement? Well, you free yourself, which is, if you like, inhibition, because freeing yourself means you stop contracting, you stop tensing. You think to be free, allow yourself to be free, and, then, you give the direction. With the freedom, then the direction, because you've got to come up. You've got to go up. You've got to have the energy to go up, and if you've got that energy there, then you will find that the breathing works for you.

You're blowing an instrument, you're singing a phrase, you're speaking, whatever it is, if you go up to do it, then the breath will be supplied. If you have doubts about it, if you think you're going to be short of breath, or you think all sorts of things that we often think in emergencies, instead of going up to breathe or sing or speak, you try and force it. You come down to do it. Now if you come down to do it, yes, you can squeeze breath out with your body, there's no difficulty about squeezing the breath out, but of course if you've squeezed it out like that then you've got quite a performance to come up again. This down and up, this up and down, is not only a waste of energy, but it's as though the race horse was going jumping forwards, going in fits and starts. It won't do. No, you've got to keep it continuously all the time.

A man called Jani Strasser was very well known as a singing coach. One of the things he used to explain to his pupils was that breathing goes on the wheel—meaning that breathing out and breathing in and breathing out and breathing in is a continuous process. You can't really say when one begins and the other finishes because they overlap.

Everybody thinks that you breathe out and then everything goes into reverse and you breathe in, and then you breathe out, and then you breathe in. It's not like that. It is like a wheel. But what keeps the wheel going? It's the continuous energy, the continuous flow of upward energy. I go up, and as I go up, that works the wheel.

Yin and yang

I WANTED TO GO ON and explain a little bit about the rib cage because when you talk about breathing, people—singing teachers, voice teachers and a lot of medical people—focus mainly on the action of the diaphragm. They mention the expansion and contraction of the rib cage but in their experience and the experience of people who deal with these things in a practical way, it is fairly rare to meet people who have much movement of the ribs. Most people are fairly stuck in the rib cage. They can do things with the ribs by making effort like throwing the shoulders back and sticking the chest out, or pulling the shoulders forward and sinking the chest in. They do specific things like that but in the ordinary way very little rib movement seems to take place.

If you look at other vertebrates, other animals, you will see that in cats, for instance, the rib cage is very mobile indeed. There is obviously a lot of movement in the ribs. It is not fixed at all. When you begin to examine the human thorax and consider how the ribs are hinged, articulated to the spine at the back, you can begin to see there is a lot of provision for movement. There is a tremendous lot of potential movement there and in accordance with our ordinary experience of using ourselves, we know that in all respects we need as much freedom and movement as we are able to obtain. We know that the tendency throughout the whole organism is towards rigidity and fixation but what is wanted for health and well-being and all the rest of it is the opposite—mobility and freedom. So there is a lot to free and a lot to observe.

When you first start teaching, you have got so much to think about and so much to see to that your observation is rather restricted. But as you get more experienced and more capable of being able to put your hands on and get the responses that you are intending, you can begin to observe more. Of course you can go through an early stage in which you hadn't noticed before, for instance, that the person was raising the shoulders or pulling the shoulder blades together when they breathed. It is very tempting at that moment, as a relatively inexperienced teacher, to point it out and say, "Don't raise your shoulders, don't narrow your back." But you find as time goes on that when you make these observations it isn't always wise to share them with the pupil straight away. You don't always want to share your discoveries immediately because you will find that the pupil promptly reacts by trying to do something about it. If you are pointing out that they are raising the shoulders, then of course they will immediately start pulling the shoulders down. If they are raising the chest then they will try and pull the chest down and do the opposite. So you have got to take all that into consideration as you continue to observe.

I was saying and explaining last time that the action of the intercostal muscles, broadly speaking, raises the ribs sideways and draws the ribs together. It generates an upward process that also produces widening and opening out. The other important feature that you have got to take into consideration is that the whole of the thorax is constructed in such a way that it is, so to speak, spring loaded to open out or expand. What I mean practically is that if you came along and cut the cartilages, the ribs coming round would spring out.

The various influences that go towards the expansion and contraction of the rib cage are very complex. You have got the action of the muscles. You have got the elasticity of the whole construction. What you actually end up with is a situation which is very well described in the Chinese terms of yin and yang. It is a counterbalance of forces. The principle of counterbalance of forces is not just a philosophical matter, it is a very practical engineering principle. By getting the counterbalance correct, you can then minimize the amount of effort and energy to be exploited to get the large effects that you need.

Breathing is something that is so finely adjusted and counterbalanced that there shouldn't be any sense of effort. You shouldn't feel that you have to make a great effort to expand in order to get more breath in or to make a great effort to expel air for singing loudly or shouting or blowing an instrument or whatever it is. The balance of forces should make it all respond very easily. Now I say "should" because it is all conditional on the one factor that people always leave out of account and overlook in ordinary voice teaching and in ordinary medical work. That is that the whole structure of the organism is designed to work on the basis of counteraction of gravitation—the upward direction of the whole organism counterbalanced by the downward action of the weight or gravitation. If these two forces, the up and the down, are not in balance then obviously the whole thing can't possibly work.

In the majority of people the overall tendency is downwards. All the structure, all the weight of the thorax, all the weight of the abdominal contents, all the weight of the liver and everything else, instead of being supported, is all being allowed to thrust downwards. With that drag and weight going down, you couldn't have a free antagonistic action that would make for effortless breathing. It isn't possible. You have to go up in order to breathe freely. This is exactly the contrary to what most people experience. Their feeling is that breathing is difficult and if it is difficult, then the remedy is to make more effort. So they make more effort and in doing so they multiply all the difficulties and make matters far worse.

Now it is recognized that somehow or another the downward pressures, the downward energy, has got to be counteracted. It is quite interesting that in the textbook here, we are looking at the action of the muscles of the neck, particularly our old friends the sternocleidomastoids. These muscles bend the neck forward when acting together and when those of one side only are acting they bend the neck to the side and turn the face towards the opposite. But they make clear in this textbook that these muscles can also act as accessory muscles of breathing like the sternomastoids. A runner in a quarter of a mile race usually finishes with the head and neck thrown well back in order to make use of these accessory muscles of respiration. So there you have the absolute official view that that is what they are good for. You throw the head well back in order to pull on those muscles. Those muscles then lift the upper part of the chest to make a bit more space and room for breathing to take place. Is this an efficient way to breathe? Absolutely not.

This same misconception about breathing holds when people have an asthma attack and are really fighting for breath. The characteristic attitude that you find adopted is that they sit with their hands on their knees, the head thrown back and the shoulders raised and they try and lift the chest by means of the arms and the shoulders and the neck muscles. They try and lift it all to try and get more breath in. Of course, all that effort doesn't achieve the result because it causes more fixation than freedom. The asthmatic during the spasm won't be able to breath until they get so exhausted and desperate that they give up the struggle. It is only when they give up the struggle trying to breath that they let the breath go out. When they let the breath go out then there is a certain amount of room for some new breath to come in. So the cycle is broken and the spasm comes to an end.

What I hope I am getting across to you is the realization that the lift of the whole structure, the mechanism that takes the whole structure up, is the mechanism that is absolutely fundamental to all breathing and all activity. If the natural mechanism that takes everything up isn't in working order, then you are in awful trouble. Whatever you try to do, whether you try to use the sternomastoids to breathe or whether you do funny things with your arms and your shoulders, it won't get you out of the trouble.

The essential requirement for all living things is the counteraction, the counterbalance of the gravitational force. As I said before, the Chinese have the words for it—the yin and the yang.

Establishing a total pattern

WE WERE TALKING recently about Professor Coghill, and we were saying he made a study of the growth and development in the nervous system, how the nerves actually grew through the body and how, at the same time, behavior developed. He was studying the two things at once through his experiments with the Amblystoma—a small lizard.

So here we are, looking at this small lizard, and the first muscular movement that is to be observed is close behind the head. Then, as growth and development takes place, the muscular contractions go further down the body, further and further along, until the entire trunk and tail are involved. And then the legs get involved in the act as part of a pattern of contraction which starts just behind the head and works throughout the body and incorporates the limbs until the little creature is actually able to make coordinated walking movements as an outcome of the working of this total pattern.

The limbs don't work separately from the trunk. That is a point that is of interest and of real practical importance to us in connection with our work and the Technique. When, for instance, people have had leg injuries, as I've had, when they've had problems in which they have to learn to walk again, all the orthopedic people, all the physios and so on, they all want to focus their attention on the limbs concerned and the musculature of the limbs. They don't take into any serious consideration what is happening throughout the length of the trunk, throughout the whole body. As Coghill's experiments demonstrated, in actual point of fact the development of the actions of the body really comes before the development of the actions of the limbs. In the beginning, the limbs act within a total pattern.

Now, in the very early stages of growth and development of the lizard, if you take a few very fine hairs, like a few hairs of a paintbrush, you produce a very interesting reaction when you touch the hairs to the skin of the lizard. In the early stages, when the skin is touched in this way, a total reaction is produced. That is to say, you can see a pattern of contraction starting behind the head and working tailwards including the limbs. It all goes pretty fast but you can nevertheless say that it starts from the head and goes tailwards. And what Coghill is saying is that, later on, when a little bit more growth and development in the nervous system has taken place, you can gently touch a limb and the leg will withdraw. It will move in response to the touch and as far as you can see there isn't any response in the rest of the musculature. The creature keeps perfectly still with no movement to be seen, except just the movement of the limb.

Now the two expressions Coghill uses to describe these events are "total pattern" and "individuation." As Coghill says about total pattern, "An action is regarded as total when it involves all the muscles of the functional system that are capable of responding at the time." A partial reaction or individuation is one in which you just appear to get the limb moving or the bit or piece or whatever moving, and nothing else.

And of course, if you look at the dissections, if you look at illustrations in anatomy books and see how the nerves grow and the way they relate to each other, indeed you can see that you're looking at a very complex pattern. This pattern of nerves is the underlying phenomenon that Coghill was looking at, as at the same time he was looking at behavior. And Coghill states it very clearly when he says, "The pattern connotes organization of the whole individual for the purposes of behavior."

Now, as far as our work is concerned, if you want deliberately to crook your little finger, of course you can do so. It is perfectly possible to make such a small movement without disturbing any other part of the body. If you want to move your hand or your foot, your arm or your leg, it is possible to move them without any disturbance of the rest of the body. But, you'll only succeed in doing that efficiently if you've got your primary control working properly—if you've got the conditions of relativity that we call primary control—that allows the freedom for an individual part to act without trouble and disturbance.

The other aspect of the situation is that if you want to move from sitting to standing, with the head leading and the body following, the legs don't work separately or independently of the whole movement. They're an integrated part of the whole movement. That is why in practical teaching, in practical work, you very often get the situation where you're trying to bring about the coordination so that the primary control is operating efficiently, and you're saying, "Don't stiffen your legs. Don't try and stand up by tightening your legs and using your legs," and they'll turn around and say to you, "Are you trying to tell me that I can stand up without using my legs?"

And it's very understandable that people get into this state of confusion, because, of course, they need to use the legs, but not in the way they think they do. After a series of lessons, the pupil gains experience in the two practical possibilities Coghill was talking about: The one is that a total pattern of action can come into play smoothly and efficiently, with the head leading and the body following. As you go to stand up, for instance, it can be a total pattern of action which is efficient and cost effective and all the rest of it. Similarly, it is possible, as in calligraphy or some delicate process of that sort, to have controlled movement of the fingertips which is very precise and exact and clearly doesn't involve movement in other parts of the body. In particular, it doesn't involve stiffening the neck and pulling the head back. So you've got the possibilities of total pattern and you've got the possibilities of partial pattern or individuation. Now individuation is obviously the result of, guess what, organized inhibition.

So here you've got a concept of inhibition, of neurological inhibition, as quite a positive nervous process, which indeed it is—when you get the individual part, the limb, the leg, just moving by itself and you don't get any other part apparently showing any response or outward signs of activity. What is going on is that the nervous system is sending inhibitory signals to all the rest saying, "No, you don't act," and just to the part that has got to act, sending a positive signal to make it act. Now, this form of neurological inhibition, or the lack of it if you like, is something that we very often see arising when people have had strokes. Because the neurological effect of a stroke very frequently is to cause a breakdown of the inhibitory process, so that muscles that you wouldn't wish to act, that are not supposed to act, will go into strong contraction because they're not being prevented from doing so. And so you get tremendous stiffness and rigidity in stroke victims because the nervous system is working in a very positive way, and bringing about this muscular activity. What is required is that somehow or another this muscular activity needs to be inhibited.

When Alexander talks about inhibition, is this the neurological inhibition we've just been speaking about? In your mind, in your thought and intent, when you say, "Now I'm not going to stiffen my neck. I'm going to move my finger, my hand or whatever, and first of all I'm giving my directions for my neck to be free and my head to go forward and up and my back to lengthen and widen." You are maintaining those directions and then going on to move your hand, and what you are doing is establishing a total pattern, which is largely in this case inhibitory. You're not going to stiffen your neck. You're not going to move this, that and the other. You establish that background pattern and then you move the bit you intend to move within that pattern.

So, Alexander's use of inhibition is very much a process of neurological inhibition. When you study the growth and development of the nervous system, and the growth and development of behavior at the same time, you see the two things are very much linked together.

Responsibility

IN THE TEACHING SITUATION, one of the
most important things of all is the matter of responsibility, the acceptance of responsibility. You could say it is
the fundamental issue. The pupil who comes, as a general rule, is unaware of the kind of responsibility that is
necessary in our work. Generally speaking, the responsibility isn't recognized, let alone acknowledged. People say
things like, "I'm not pulling myself down, gravity is
pulling me down," or, "My back just started hurting, I
didn't do anything." There are always lots and lots of
explanations as to why things have happened, but there
comes a time when you have got to acknowledge your
own responsibility in the matter.

But you don't get people to acknowledge responsibility
by talking to them about it; that is certainly not going to
help. The starting point is you've got to face your own
responsibility. You've got to face your responsibility to
yourself. That's exactly what the work that we do in the
training course is all about. We do emphasize all the time
that the first requirement is to look after yourself. You've
got to be responsible for yourself and look after yourself

and that continues just as much when you're teaching. So you're responsible for yourself. You are, of course, also responsible for your pupil. You may say this is quite a weight of responsibility and so it is, but this is where the Technique comes in, because since we do have a practical technique, we do have a practical way of coping with the responsibility and enabling our pupils to come round to recognizing and acknowledging their own responsibility.

First and foremost it is up to you to give them, as well as you can, the good experience of non-interference, of lightness and freedom—the experience of going up rather than pulling down. The experience that you give them in that way is a novel and unfamiliar experience. People don't necessarily like it at first. It comes as a surprise. It comes as quite a shock. The experience needs to be repeated and repeated and you can't expect them to understand it or assimilate it all at once. It's going to take quite a lot of time before they begin to understand it and begin to real-ize the significance of it. And out of the experience and the understanding will come gradually this recognition of responsibility. The pupil will find out, as you have found out, that it is up to them to say no, or up to them to say yes. It's up to them to direct or not to direct. It is up to them to find out what they really want and not to try to kid themselves or anybody else that they want things that they don't want. Because for them, as for you, if you try and persuade yourself that you want things that you don't want, then you will get into trouble.

And one of the things that makes this responsibility so hard to take is that we are creatures of habit in our thought and in our feeling, in our reaction, in every sort of way, and so, to a very large extent, we are really not free. We can kid ourselves that we are free. We like to think that we are free. In actual point of fact, all our friends and relations can observe and point out that our reactions are habitual, predictable and certainly not the outcome of any process of rational choice and decision. They are more the outcome of habit. But if you can manage to do something to change habit, to intervene and control the habitual response, then indeed freedom in thought and action does become a reality. Then you really do have some choice in how you react and really what mental attitude, what patterns of thought, you adopt in connection with all the different things that come up. But it's only if you're able to exert control of habit, of choice in the matter, that you've got any chance of freedom.

Gravitation

THE RESPONSE OF ANY living thing to gravitation is absolutely of fundamental importance. The less effectively any living thing responds to gravitation, the worse it is going to function, and the more trouble it is going to have. In life, we need air to breathe, we need food to eat, but you need the effective response to gravitation or you are not going to stay alive.

Under conditions of daily life, we get ourselves out of balance. We get ourselves discoordinated and develop habits of muscular contraction for all kinds of reasons— not only the obvious mechanical reasons, but for emotional reasons as well. These reactions express themselves in muscle tension of one sort or another. Once muscles have contracted on that habitual basis, it isn't an easy matter, it certainly isn't an instantaneous matter by any means, to get them all to lengthen out and free and come into shape again.

Now the big problem is whether we can perceive the interference kinesthetically. But you will remember this is what we were reading yesterday in *Man's Supreme Inheritance.* Alexander put debauched kinesthesia, as he called it, at the head of the list. So what he was really saying was that you are going to have quite a hard time perceiving the interference kinesthetically. Oftentimes, you don't really notice what you are doing to yourself. You don't notice the tension you are making. It doesn't register. Since it is apt to be painful and uncomfortable, you don't particularly want it to register. You try to ignore it, and one of the best ways of messing up the kinesthetic register is to ignore it.

I had a little instance of this at the weekend. I was giving an old pupil of mine a lesson and her girlfriend, who knew nothing about the Technique, came along and watched as I gave the lesson. I tried to explain a little bit of what I was doing and so forth and at the end of it I said to her, "Well would you just like me to show you. Would you just like to see for yourself," and so rather hesitantly she said she would. And so I got her standing there and I got her looking out of the window and just seeing what there was to be seen. She left herself alone and I was able to correct her balance and straighten her out a bit and she said, "Good gracious, that is amazing. It has taken all the strain out of my back." I said "Yes, I expect it has, but the way you were sitting a few minutes ago, that was what you were doing to your back. If you do that to your back you have got to expect that you feel strain."

That is the message about kinesthesia. She had been sitting there listening to me and watching and so on, but she hadn't felt at all. It hadn't registered kinesthetically what she was doing to herself. That was completely ignored. It hadn't penetrated to her consciousness. But when she let me put a hand on her, then she suddenly began to feel what was going on and she correctly felt then that by straightening out and coming into balance, she was taking the pressure off. So kinesthetic perception is absolutely critical, because if you can feel what is going on, you have got a possibility of stopping. If you can't feel what is going on, you haven't got a hope in hell of stopping it.

By means of stopping the interference, by means of stopping the wrong thing, the anti-gravity response is facilitated. The anti-gravity response is facilitated by thinking the right thoughts and bringing yourself into the correspondingly balanced attitude. People still have some vague idea that in order to go up you have got to do something. You give the orders, you say, "Neck to be free, head forward and up," but there is an idea that you have got to do something. Of course doing involves muscular contraction which is entirely counterproductive. No, you don't have to do something, but you do have to see that something actually happens. The anti-gravity response is an absolutely genuine thing that happens. It takes place. It is a happening. That is what it is. It is not a doing, it is a happening. It is a happening that is facilitated by your wishes and your thoughts and your observation, particularly your kinesthetic observation.

Through your kinesthesia you feel tension, you feel stiffness, you feel that things are wrong, so on that basis you try and cut it out, you try and avoid it and then the change can happen. Of course when it does happen, it very definitely does have an integrative effect on the organism. It is going to stimulate the breathing because as soon as you do get the anti-gravity response, as we all know from experience, you feel a release and the breathing suddenly begins to free. In the same way, although you may not feel it, because you are not squashing the veins and arteries, circulation is easier. You have expanded and opened out the thorax, so while you were freeing the breathing, you were giving the heart more room to work. You were also taking pressure off the whole digestive apparatus. What it amounts to quite simply is that you are facilitating, helping, encouraging better general functioning.

Bear in mind that if you use the expression general functioning, you mustn't expect people to understand what you are talking about. The concept of general functioning doesn't exist in medical science. It isn't something that they take on board at all. The functioning of the heart yes, the functioning of this system or that system, the functioning of this bit or that bit, is understood very well and in very considerable detail. If you then mention general functioning, the response you would most likely get is that it is the sum of all the bits. You take all the separate bits and put them together and that is general functioning. But of course it isn't at all. The whole is more than the sum of the parts because of the integrative action of the anti-gravity response that we have just been talking about. Because if you haven't got a satisfactory response to gravitation then inevitably all the separate aspects of functioning will suffer—some in a greater and some in a lesser degree. With different individuals it will probably be different, but you can say that if you get the anti-gravity response improved, then they will all improve.

Saying and meaning no

WHEN YOU HAVE SOMEBODY standing in
front of a chair and the idea is that they are being asked
to sit, they should say "No." Instead of them proceeding
to send the messages to carry out the habitual procedure
that is called "sitting down," they should say "No," and
send messages to the neck to be free and the head to go
forward and up and so on. They are attempting, with
your help, to bring about a quite different procedure
from their normal habitual one. This changed thought
and movement involves, among other things, releasing
the knees so that gravity takes them into the chair and, at
the same time, the balancing mechanism works properly
so that in letting the knees go they don't lose their balance and they go into the chair lightly and freely without
a bump. That is, of course, what is wanted.

Even when the pupil understands this and is clear
about this in their minds—they know what they want,
they know what messages they've got to give and all the
rest of it—somehow it doesn't seem to work out.
Alexander describes this as trying to be right. He says
that you have the fairly strong stimulus of wanting to do

what you are supposed to do, wanting to carry out the teacher's instructions, and if you are going to try to carry out the teachers instructions and do what you are supposed to do, you will inevitably be guided by your feelings and you will do what feels to be the proper thing to do in order to gain success. You'll do what feels to be right in the circumstances. This is what is going to get you into trouble.

Research and study of the nervous system and the neuromuscular system have come up with information that really casts quite an important light on all of this. Before you are consciously aware that you're actually going to make a movement—for example, a movement from standing to sitting—your nervous system at some earlier point and on some subconscious level has already got hold of the idea. In response to that idea, the neuro-muscular system has started to activate a habitual pattern of action so that events are taking place in your nerves and your muscles in a habitual pattern that is normally used for sitting down. You haven't realized that you've got the intention of sitting. You might say you haven't even thought of sitting, but in fact your body has gone quite a long way in the process.

Now at a certain point you do become aware you are going to sit and at this point you say, "No, I don't want to sit, or at least what I want is, I want my neck to be free and I want my head to go forward and up and I want to go up not down." You think and direct that but it does not work out because in actual fact you have gone too far along the old familiar habitual path. You really are, without realizing it, already committed to acting in the old habitual way. You do not seem able to stop at that point. What you don't realize is that the reason it is so difficult to stop is that you've not only started but you are already quite a long way into the process.

If you are going to stop effectively, it's got to be a very positive realization of what is going on and the "No" has got to be a very definite "No," so that no way are you going to persist or going to have anything to do with the whole business of going down or bending your knees or any of those things. You're not going to do anything like that. What you are going to do is something that is utterly and totally different. If you can make this inhibition really effective in that way and stop off the old habitual pattern, then you have got the possibility of being able to generate a new pattern and get things working in a different way, in a way that you have chosen and a way that you want.

Of course, this will take time. It will not be quick and it will not be easy. There will be a lot of uncertainty in it because the new way is going to be unfamiliar. Until you actually try and get into it you haven't got the experience to know what it is really and truly like and what it involves. It doesn't solve all the problem—you have effectively choked off the old but you've still got a tremendous lot to deal with to generate the new. What

Alexander is saying and what we all find in teaching is that until you have effectively choked off the old, until you have really learned what inhibition means in that way, you're not going to get any further and make the change that you want.

Any experienced teacher has this demonstrated every day. You've got a pupil standing in front of the chair and you say, "Now I'm going to ask you to sit down and I don't want you to do it, I want you to say, 'No.' Instead of sitting down I want you to think of your neck being free and your head going forward and up," and so on. You go through this explanation but you can feel with your hand and you can see that the pupil hasn't inhibited, or they haven't inhibited effectively, and whatever directions they may have given about freeing the neck and going up, at the back of their mind, they are thinking of the chair and they are thinking of going down. You can see this and you can feel it and so you can be absolutely sure that it is going wrong until you intervene and help in some way to get them to inhibit and stop off the habitual preparation. The energy is there to make it work, all of the stuff that the neurologists call the "readiness potential" is there. All systems are at "go," but it is all pointing in the wrong direction. The energy is going in the wrong direction: "Go" pointing down instead of "Go" pointing up, you see.

It is people's feelings that matter and these feelings involve, "I'm going to do something. I'm going to move.

I wonder if I can do it this time. I think I'm going to fail again. I'm going to make a mess of it once more." These are the sorts of feelings that are attached to it and they are mostly anxious feelings. You are really saying to people that it is not only saying, "No" to the movement but it is "No" to all these sorts of feelings, calming yourself, getting your thoughts and feelings together in such a way that no longer are you so involved in trying to gain this end.

What you are striving for, of course, is that the pupil no longer be subconsciously or otherwise entertaining the idea of sitting down. When you are able to get the pupil calm enough to accomplish this, you can then go on to encourage the pupil to very positively and very consciously project the idea of leaving himself alone and not trying to do anything. That is the condition that makes it possible for the teacher to introduce new and different experiences and to open up the possibility of a different way. But you can only introduce a pupil to the new pathway when they absolutely finally abandon trying to follow the old pathway. Then they are entirely ready and open to be shown and to be led.

This isn't a short journey. They may reach that point after one hundred and fifty lessons, something of this sort. It is a long and difficult job to get them to this point, to get them to stop trying, to stop them from making the effort in the wrong direction. But that is what the job is. That is the essence of the matter.

A *sense of insecurity*

As HUMAN BEINGS walking around on two feet, performing our rather brilliant balancing act, the normal situation is to be light, to be free, unaware that you are performing a balancing act, unaware that there is any instability or any threat to your stability. But when something happens in life that causes this to be upset, then you start using yourself in a different way. If your balance is not working correctly, then obviously you are in danger of falling over if you do not do something about it. What you do about it is you make tension somewhere or another. You increase the muscle tension in order to make yourself more secure. Holding yourself, even though it is for a perfectly sensible reason of seeking security, is misuse.

This misuse becomes associated with all sorts of feelings. Take bracing your knees back, for instance. You want to be able to stand on your feet and stand upright without the least danger of falling over, so you brace your knees back. Bracing your knees back is a form of misuse because by doing so you sacrifice mobility and fluidity. There is no question that braced knees are an abnormal condition. At the same time, it comes to be associated with a feeling of security, so the stiffness and relative awkwardness that you feel as you brace the knees back come to feel acceptable because you associate them with security. In ideal conditions, under normal conditions, bracing of the knees might feel quite wrong because you would rightly realize that bracing interferes with mobility and fluid movement.

If you can manage to change people's use, which is always a big if, but if you can manage to do it and get them to accept what is involved in change, then you are certainly on the way to making an important change in eradicating the abnormality. But it is asking quite a lot of people. You're asking people to risk their sense of security, to run the risk of feeling insecure, of feeling a loss of control, of confronting the unknown.

In good use, the basic proposition is that you want to move lightly and freely and not fall over. In good use, muscular effort is at all times economized and reduced to a minimum. That does not mean to say that when circumstances demand it strength is not available and strength is not used. There are many situations in life where strength is called for and has got to be used, but obviously if you are going to use strength you want to ensure that you use it in as productive a manner as possible—in other words, that you get the best return for the amount of strength that you put out. You don't want to waste any of it. Economy of effort means exactly what it says. It means that the amount of effort is proportional to the requirement, to the job in hand. This is not what we are taught from a very early age. Children are taught to make more effort, more muscular effort, and more effort of all kinds, and oftentimes really for the sake of making effort.

From the point of view of our education and our general way of carrying on, you would think that there is a positive virtue in making more effort. In fact some people think that there is. They think that to make little effort is somehow morally wrong or morally suspect. The virtuous thing is to get busy and make as much effort as possible. If you are educated on those lines, if that is what you are encouraged to do from the time you are small, your use of yourself will deteriorate progressively. In everything you do you will be using yourself in such a way that you are making greater and greater effort.

As people go on making tension, they get used to unnecessary levels of tension and muscular effort. They get used to levels of stress that affect the breathing mechanism and the circulatory system. As you have heard me say very often, people go around trying to squeeze the life out of themselves. You can go around for a long time busily squeezing the life out of yourself until you squeeze to a point where suddenly something goes pop. Squeezing for many people seems natural and comforting. The idea is that you are getting your act together, you're getting a grip on yourself. That's how it works and then the grip goes on to a point where something suddenly goes pop and than you say, "Oh, this problem just came out of the blue. It was totally unexpected."

When you stop your pupils from squeezing the life out of themselves, they can feel so insecure. It is always well to remember that your pupils are giving up a lot to make these changes. Many of them will have been reinforcing these attitudes their entire lives. You are working to reverse the process of squeezing the life out, and that is a very foreign, often unsettling, experience. Your pupils really do need quite a lot of care and sympathetic consideration. It is your job to nurse them over the very unpleasant sensory experiences that they are liable to get in the course of ultimately coming around to greater freedom and, hopefully, to something more like true happiness.

Change without changing

In life there's a great deal that people would prefer to ignore and not be conscious of. People really don't very much want to be conscious a lot of the time. We talk these days quite a lot about changes of consciousness and how by drugs and narcotics and various things of one sort or another you can change consciousness. But the fundamental problem is that the majority of people are not all that keen on being conscious, fully conscious, all the time. Consciousness can definitely seem to be too painful.

I remember an old pupil of mine who was in quite a high position in an insurance company. He was known for being very conservative, very, very staid, very conventional. I was giving him a lesson one day and he said, "You know, a groove is a very comfortable thing." And he was expressing, quite obviously, a deep feeling that he was having. He realized that in the work I was doing I was trying to winkle him out of his groove, and he didn't want to be winkled out of that. He wanted to be able to pursue his course of life as before. He didn't want to change.

And on the whole, people don't want to change. They're very, very, very reluctant to change. They come, of course, for lessons on the understanding that this method is going to open up a way for them to change, but the change that they want is a change in which everything can remain the same. They want to change without changing. They haven't got the actual experience of what change is like. When they actually get the experience of it, most people are rather frightened of it, and certainly they don't like it. And so they adopt all sorts of defenses and affectations and evasions and so on that as a teacher you've got to battle with and work your way round if you're going to keep the impetus to change. And I'm speaking of change now in the wider and general sense of consciousness and conscious awareness.

In all of these attempts at change, it is essential to keep in mind that the challenge for change is with the physical aspect of your self—it is your breathing and your circulation and your digestion. It's the habits attached to your postural mechanism, to your muscular habits. And then, even more important than muscular habits are your neurological habits, because all the nerve pathways and all the inter-connections whereby energy flows from one nerve center to another are very largely habitual. The energy flows along habitual lines. It's like water running in an irrigation system in fields. It runs along habitual lines because those lines have become so familiar. That is how the energy flows.

Now, we are seeking to change people's manner of use of themselves. We are seeking to bring about changes not merely in their thought and their feelings on the larger scale—their habits, their social habits, and all that side of it, all the side I was referring to with the man from the insurance company—but also the absolutely personal habits insofar as it affects the use of the self and the whole working of the neuromuscular system. And to change all that, to begin to change it, to begin to make any change, any impression on it, is really quite an undertaking. It's a pretty daunting task as you can see when you see how much there is to be changed.

But imagine if somebody doesn't want to change, if they are really against change, afraid of it. You've got a hard task on your hands. It is a hard task. But to have any chance at success, you have to look at how people use themselves. You are not going to be able to make a significant change in yourself or in others until you address the whole problem of how people use themselves. That is really the crux of this whole business.

The act of living

FROM A PRACTICAL POINT of view, from a practical teaching point of view, you will find that you do come up against people who have the egotism to believe that things are of their doing. This is not just a philosophical or theoretical consideration, it's an absolutely practical one when it comes to trying to help people to make change. On more than one occasion, I've said to someone, "Now, I don't want you to do anything," and they turn around with perfect seriousness and say, "But if I don't do anything, I shall fall down." They do have the absolute fundamental belief that if they don't do something, then nothing will happen. Everything that goes on depends on their doing.

I'm afraid that education, certainly in the past, the attitude of parents and teachers, used to be very, very much on those lines: You've got to try harder. You've got to make more effort. You've got to do it. You mustn't just dream and think about it, you've got to get out there and do it. That sort of attitude leads to the egotistic belief in the end that everything depends on their doing. Since people have this belief, and really they do have it deeply ingrained in them, if you challenge that belief or give them anything to make them realize that this might be incorrect, it does arouse anxiety, if not fear.

So, in moving from the situation in which they're trying hard to stand up and trying hard to put the head forward and up, trying hard to lengthen, they perhaps finally are able to stop doing or reduce the doing, but what comes out of this change is a state of anxiety. Anxiety expresses itself as a disturbance of the breathing rhythm specifically, and an overall pulling down generally. So, if you're teaching somebody, you've got to be very careful how you challenge these ideas. Yes, you want them to stop trying to do the work for you, but it is up to you to watch very, very closely the reactions you get from the pupil. It is very important for teachers to remember that if you get the wrong reaction, from your point of view, the chances are not that it's the pupil's fault, but that it's your fault. The odds are very likely that you have given the wrong stimulus.

You've got to work with people for a long time before you are justified in believing in the possibility that they don't react to stimulus. Everybody reacts to stimulus. They react to stimulus along habitual lines. If you know that your pupil is going to react along those lines, then isn't it your fault if you give them the wrong stimulus? You've pressed the wrong button, so who is responsible when you get the wrong result? You've only got yourself to blame.

And just as the teaching situation can get unnecessarily encumbered, so, too, can life in general get needlessly complicated. As Alexander pointed out, people can unnecessarily complicate the act of living. We don't usually speak of the act of living. You're alive, and you live. But the idea that living is an act, that living is something that we undertake, that goes on, helps you realize that you'd better set about living it and see what's involved in living it. It truly is an act of living. It may seem like a fine wire balancing act between not trying to do, not having the egotism to believe if you don't do something, nothing will happen, and on the other hand, the realization that living is an act. But if you think further, you will see it isn't a contradiction. Both go on at once. Living is an act, and in this act, we all too easily allow our activities to be encumbered and encrusted with habits, with conventions, with all kinds of complicated influences.

And in the act of living, whether it is walking down the street or learning to play the piano, you must keep in mind that the primary energy cost is the support of the body weight. If the body weight is not being supported efficiently, then there is a tremendous energy leak, and the whole process of living will not be efficient. That is what the pupil is faced with, that is what we are faced with in ourselves. We need to learn to reduce the interference that is causing that tremendous lot of vital energy being dissipated. That is where doing less, inhibition, comes in. So without any doubt at all, you've got to recognize that in living, in learning, the efficient working not only of the physical side, not only of the mental side, not only of the nervous system, but the standard of functioning of the whole lot must be maintained at a high level. When you've got to that point, it won't seem such a contradiction any more. When you've got to that point, you've come up to the starting gate and you're ready to take off. But not until then.

Biographies

Walter Carrington was born in 1915, the only child of the Rev. W.M. and Hannah Carrington. He was educated in the Choir School of All Saints, Margaret St., London and St. Paul's School. He first had lessons with Mr. Alexander in 1935 and joined his Training Course in 1936, qualifying as a teacher of the Technique in 1939. From 1941 to 1946 he served as a pilot in the Royal Air Force, after which he returned to work as an Assistant Teacher, and then carried on the Training Course after Mr. Alexander's death in 1955. He and his wife Dilys were Directors of the Constructive Teaching Centre Ltd in London and he was a past Chairman of the Society of Teachers of the Alexander Technique (S.T.A.T.). He died August 7th, 2005, at the age of 90.

Glynn Macdonald has taught the Alexander Technique for twenty-five years. She is a past Secretary and Chairman of The Society of Teachers of the Alexander Technique (S.T.A.T.). She has taught in the major English drama and music schools and has lectured throughout the world. Her television and radio appearances include *Back to Work* for the BBC, *Does He Take Sugar, Woman's Hour* and *The Time, The Place* and *Saturday Morning* for CBS. She works at Shakespeare's Globe in London, and has written *The Complete Illustrated Guide to Alexander Technique,* published by Element Books and Barnes and Noble.

Mistakenly selected, when young, for specialization in mathematics, **Tris Roberts** found himself, before the war, working in a Life Assurance Office and training, unsuccessfully, to become an actuary. The war brought a sharp change in direction, as he worked for a time in the accounts office of a hospital and studying at Chelsea Polytechnic in the evenings for a combined honours degree in Zoology, Physiology and Chemistry. During a first year (1946/7) as a graduate student in the Zoology Department at Edinburgh, he was invited to join Otto Lowenstein in the Glasgow Zoology Department to work on the neurophysiology of the otolith organs in the skate. In 1950, he was asked to set up experimental neurophysiology in the Physiology Department also at Glasgow. Thereafter, his lifetime study became the role of the labyrinth and other proprioceptors in balance, posture and locomotion in man and other animals.

Dr. Tris Roberts is the author of three books: *Neurophysiology of Postural Mechanisms,* London: Butterworth. (1967, 2nd Ed. 1978); *Understanding Balance,* London: Chapman & Hall, 1995 (A completely revised assessment of the evidence presented in *NPM* above); and *Equestrian Technique*, London: J.A. Allen, 1992 (a textbook based on a distillation of the writings of the classical masters of equitation, with explanatory appendices, reflecting a lifetime extramural interest). He has written numerous papers and three teaching films. His hobbies, in historical order, include: gliding (pre-war only), dinghy sailing, swimming, squash (all now more or less discontinued), horse riding, and scientific writing (both still active).

Jerry Sontag is publisher and editor of Mornum Time Press. Mornum Time Press specializes in books on education. Jerry is also a teacher of the Alexander Technique, having trained at the Center for the Alexander Technique in Menlo Park, California from 1982 through 1985. Jerry runs an Amsat certified teacher training program, and has a private teaching practice in Berkeley, California.

THIS BOOK WAS DESIGNED AND PRODUCED on the Macintosh using Quark Xpress. The text is set in Bembo. Bembo was modeled on typefaces cut by Francesco Griffo for Aldus Manutius' printing of De Aetna in 1495 in Venice, a book by classicist Pietro Bembo about his visit to Mount Etna. Griffo's design is considered one of the first of the old style typefaces, which include Garamond, that were used as staple text types in Europe for 200 years. Bembo italic is modeled on the handwriting of the Renaissance scribe Giovanni Tagliente.